BIRTH AND
OUR BODIES

The Author

Paddy O'Brien was born in 1953 in Gateshead. She now lives in Southampton and is a lecturer in the history of art and design. She has practised and taught yoga for many years and also teaches self-defence and assertiveness. For the past few years she has run active birth classes and seminars at local maternity hospitals and has just opened Active Birth South, a centre for women approaching and coming through pregnancy, labour and birth. She has three children, and wrote this book while expecting her fourth.

The Illustrator

Susan Hartley was born in 1936 in Hertfordshire. She now lives in Southampton. For many years she worked as a university lecturer and taught human biology to medical students. She is now a freelance writer and illustrator, recording areas of women's lives today which are not usually properly recorded in our society; the reality of childbirth is a powerful example of this. Susan has three children.

Good luck with it!

PANDORA PRESS HANDBOOK

For a list of books in this series, see the end of the book.

BIRTH AND OUR BODIES

PADDY O'BRIEN
Illustrated by Susan Hartley

Exercises and

Meditations for the

Childbearing Year

and Preparation

for Active Birth

London

First published in 1986
by Pandora Press
(Routledge & Kegan Paul plc)

11 New Fetter Lane, London EC4P 4EE

Set in Palatino
by Columns, Reading
and printed in Great Britain
by The Guernsey Press Co Ltd
Guernsey, Channel Islands

British Library Cataloguing in Publication Data
O'Brien, Paddy
Birth and our bodies: exercises and meditation for the
childbearing year and preparation for active birth.—
(Pandora handbook)
1. Exercises for women 2. Pregnancy
I. Title.
613.7'1   RG558.7
ISBN 0-86358-047-5 (pbk)

This book is dedicated to all women
considering pregnancy and approaching birth.

CONTENTS

FIGURES

FIGURES

ACKNOWLEDGMENTS

My thanks are due to all the women who have come to my active birth classes and shared so much of what they have thought, felt and experienced during their pregnancies and labours. I'd also like to thank my yoga teachers over the years: Penny Nields-Smith, Betty Davis, Linda Hayes and Verena Poole; and various people whose workshops and classes have been inspirational: Khofi Busia, Mel Huxley, Jonathan Kaye and Anna Room.

I'd like to thank Susan Hartley, my illustrator, for drawing classes and births with such understanding, and rushing out on her bike in horrible weather to draw births when necessary!

Norma Appleton and Sara Roch of the Princess Anne Maternity Hospital in Southampton have always given the greatest support and encouragement, and have been sources of expert knowledge, and Glenys Fairclough and Marion Symes have been patient and full of good humour whenever I've needed it. Lorraine Curtis and Sue Cavanagh, also of the Princess Anne Maternity Hospital, have been the consultant midwives at the class for many months and their help has always been greatly appreciated.

Lyndis Pursey and Maggie Harrison, both health visitors, have been enthusiastic and supportive in the community. Lastly, thanks to Tim, Jonathan, Benjamin and Daniel.

WHAT YOU CAN FIND IN THIS BOOK

Becoming pregnant, carrying and then giving birth to your baby is a series of exciting and difficult experiences. This book suggests physical exercises, massages, meditations and counselling exercises to help you to explore, and grow, in more ways than the obvious one, through these moving times.

Exercise is a way of staying in touch, and friends, with your body as it goes through the changes of pregnancy, birth and recovery. It can also be a way of staying in charge of your body when it seems in danger of being taken over by your baby, or by the doctors and midwives with whom you come into contact.

If you make these exercises a part of your life you will maintain and strengthen your muscles, especially those, like your abdominals and pelvic floor muscles, which are in for maximum stress and stretch. As you get stronger and more supple physically you become stronger and more supple emotionally – so it's easier to handle the joy, tenderness, pain, tiredness and other intensities of pregnancy, birth and life with a new baby.

The book works chronologically through from the time before your baby is conceived up until she is 3 months old. As you approach birth you will have built up quite a range of exercises with which you're familiar. After your baby is born you add a few more to aid recovery, to stay comfortable while full of milk, and to help accustom your abdomen to its new state.

If you don't pick this book up until you're 6 or 7 months pregnant, don't worry – read through the early chapters and work out the stretches and exercises described there, and then start spending some time on the 6-9 months chapter. There's still time to make quite a difference to how fit you feel and how your birth goes.

Only *you* can give birth to *your* baby. Each of us realizes and works on this revelation as and when we can. Some women feel it from the moment of conception, others find out as the baby starts kicking, others in the few days before birth, others not until the middle of labour! If you can start to absorb that amazing, and perhaps frightening fact as you learn your stretches and breathing, you are allowing your mind as well as your body to get itself ready. And to learn how special your particular body, your particular baby, and your rhythms together, can be.

The exercises described in this book are particularly useful if you want to get ready for an active birth, where you will hope to keep moving around during your labour, rocking and swaying your hips through contractions, to use little or no painkillers, and to push your baby out squatting, or kneeling, or on all fours. But you may choose, or in an emergency you may need, an epidural anaesthetic, or even a Caesarean section. If this happens, don't feel you have wasted your time. A fit and supple body recovers more readily from surgery. Women who have worked out how to release their pelvic floors and push are often able to push their babies out even with an epidural anaesthetic (which makes you numb from waist to feet) without forceps or a tear. Also, an emotional flexibility comes with physical confidence, and can help to make any frightening or unhappy moments in your labour more manageable.

Making a tape of the exercises you need for your particular phase would be a good way of using this book. Read the instructions for each stretch or exercise clearly and slowly on to the tape and leave yourself a few seconds to complete each exercise. When an exercise is mentioned several times in the book it is described in detail the first time and more briefly later on. When you make your tape always look up and read out the most detailed instructions. Then, when you come to the next 3 month phase you can erase your tape and put the next set of exercises on to it.

Do your exercises in loose clothing in a warm, cleared space. Check first with your GP or midwife that there is no reason, diabetes or high blood pressure for example, why you should not exercise steadily and sensibly by yourself. If you do ever feel any strain, stop at once, and take up one of the relaxation positions. Forget about 'working hard', 'discipline' and 'getting it right': think instead about awarding yourself the time and space to get to know about yourself, your baby, and the birth you are going to go through together.

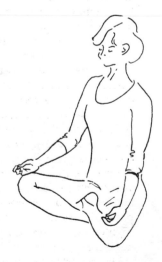

Sitting introspecting – take time to find your own quiet place

CHAPTER 1

BEFORE THE BEGINNING:

EXERCISES FOR PRE-CONCEPTION

Conception doesn't always happen exactly when we want it to. Indeed, there is some evidence that the more couples worry about it, the less likely they are to conceive. We vary so much: for some couples fertility ticks away constantly like a time bomb and they have to put a huge effort into avoiding it; others wait months or even years for a conception. Nevertheless if you feel you'd like to conceive during the next few months you can begin to prepare your body.

Firstly, try to evolve a sensible, everyday diet high in raw fruit and vegetables, brown bread, baked potatoes, and pulses (i.e. beans and lentils), low in sugar, and lowish in fat. Try to phase out cigarettes, and try to get out of the habit of bingeing on alcohol or relying on tranquillisers. Have a glass of wine now and again in the evening by all means, but otherwise get in the habit of drinking fruit juices and mineral waters. It's only the first few weeks without chocolate bars, lunchtime booze or cigarettes that are tough. You won't believe it at first, but it's true that once you've taught your body to expect decent food and a lack of poisons such as nicotine it genuinely prefers it. The point of doing this before you conceive is not only that it's really good for your baby to start off in as healthy an environment inside you as possible, but also that it's far easier to grapple with giving up smoking or sorting your eating habits out if you're not coping with the early stages of pregnancy as well!

If it looks as though you're going to have a long wait for your baby (if your periods turn up with that disappointing low stomach ache month after month), don't lose heart. Do your exercises as casually as you can, almost pretending it has nothing to do with babies; perhaps join an ordinary yoga class too. These are the best exercises for pre-conception. They increase strength and suppleness and enhance relaxation. They should help you to be comfortable and receptive to conception.

Read the following exercises once through slowly, then try them out one by one with the book next to you. In a few days they'll become quite familiar.

HEAD, NECK AND SHOULDERS

Sit cross-legged on the floor. If your knees feel very stiff uncross your legs and push your feet away from you a bit so your knees flop outwards, but not too much.

Pull your bottom backwards a bit with your hands to make sure you are sitting on the centre of your pelvic floor.

Now stretch your spine upwards; lift the crown of your head towards the ceiling. Release your shoulders down. You're like an arrow: the spine lifts upwards, your shoulders relax downwards. Have a sense of your spine as a strong, flexible stalk, your head balanced on top like a flower.

Breathing steadily, remind yourself this is your own time. If distractions and worries intrude on your mind, collect them all together, take a deep breath in, and on the breath out, start to breathe them away. On the breath in, breathe in peace – on the breath out, breathe out tension. In the rhythm of your own breathing continue to centre yourself in this way as long as you feel you want to.

Then, when you're steady, start to make deep stretches in your neck and shoulders.

Breathe in; lift your spine up; breathing out, slowly drop your chin forward on to your chest. Linking your hands, place them on the back of your head; let your elbows relax down so your arms lie along the sides of your forehead. Keep your spine lifting and experience the stretch in your upper back and the back of your neck. Keep breathing steadily.

After 30 seconds or so, on a breath in release your hold and rest your hands on your knees. Let your head float up; on the breath out let it release back so the crown of your head stretches down towards the floor behind you. Take your lower lip over your upper lip a few times to stretch your throat. On a breath in float your head back up; on the breath out stretch your right ear towards your right shoulder. Experience the stretch in the left side of your neck. Breathe steadily in an ordinary rhythm.

After 15 seconds or so, on a breath in float your head up; on the breath out release it down, left ear to left shoulder. This time feel the right side of your neck stretch. After about 15 seconds, on a breath in let your head rise again. On a breath out look over your right shoulder. Breathe in, breathe out, look a fraction further. Breathe in, and on the breath out come back to the centre. Now do this on the other side. Check that your spine is lifting, your shoulders relaxed.

At first all this spine-lifting is a struggle, but soon it feels quite natural that your spine flies upwards from its base deep in the back of your pelvis. Think how this frees your central nervous system, housed in the core of your spine. Think how it will help when your baby starts to grow inside you and alters your balance.

FIGURE 1.1

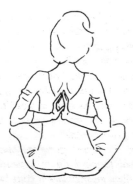

Hands behind back – to open out your chest

Now, if possible, lifting your spine, put your hands palm to palm behind your back (Figure 1.1) and stretch your upper chest. Be aware of the muscles under your breasts. They need to stretch and tone because your breasts will get heavier. If your hands won't go palm to palm, hold opposite elbows, or opposite wrists, still feeling the stretch in the upper chest. Do whatever's right for you on that particular day. In yoga there's no competition, no prize. The work that you do is just for you.

FIGURE 1.2

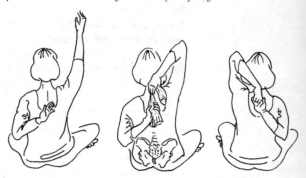

Hands, socks, held behind back, three types

Hold that stretch for 30 seconds, breathing steadily, then slowly release it. Now work your left hand up between your shoulder blades. Make sure you're sitting tall. Breathe in and stretch your right hand straight up in the air then, breathing out, bend it at the elbow and try to make contact with your left hand (Figure 1.2). If it won't reach, hold the end of a sock or scarf or anything suitable in either hand. Keep breathing gently and hold the stretch for 20 seconds or so. Breathing in, release and stretch your right hand up. On your breath out glide it down to your side. Sitting tall, do the stretch on the other side, with your right hand between your shoulder blades and your left hand reaching up then bending and stretching down to your right fingertips.

After doing these simple and effective stretches even for five or six days in a row you will notice a strength and suppleness coming. Once you have faith in one lot of muscles growing stronger and stretchier it is easy to see how all the other muscles which need to be stretchy and strong for pregnancy and birth can be greatly helped with your yoga practice.

STANDING, SIDEWAYS AND FORWARD STRETCHES

Just as you can sit to make more space in the front of your body by sitting on the centre of your pelvic floor, so you can stand to make more room in the front of the body. In yoga it is considered so important to stand well that there is a posture simply devoted to just that. It is called 'tadasana' or 'mountain pose'.

Stand with your feet together, big toe joints and ankles lined up. Starting from the soles of your feet get a sense of everything in your body lifting upwards, except your shoulders (and eyebrows!) which relax downwards. Let your spine fly up. Now tuck your tailbone in: this way you scoop all your pelvic organs upwards and inwards, not slopping them forwards on to your abdominal muscles. Relax your hands by your sides. Lift the crown of your head. Experience that way of standing for a few moments. Now allow yourself to stand as though you were very tired or depressed. Notice the difference. Come back to standing in mountain pose. Notice how it gives you confidence and strength to stand this way.

Without losing the feeling of standing in that special way (it's also called the 'fearless pose'), step your feet 3-3½ feet apart and turn your left foot in, your right foot out. Look to see that your right heel is in line with your left instep. Breathing in, lift your arms out to the side at shoulder level. Breathing out, release your shoulders and stretch your fingertips out. Breathing in once more, wait; breathing out, reach out as far as you can to the right, then release down to the right place for you (Figure 1.3). Don't bend forwards in order to come further down. Look at the upper thumb with the lower eye and keep breathing. Keep your face and throat relaxed. At first you will only want to hold this stretch for 5-10 seconds. After a while you will settle into it for much longer. When you feel it's right for you, on a breath in come up, and breathing out, release your arms down. Now make the whole stretch again the other way. This is called 'trikonasana' or

FIGURE 1.3

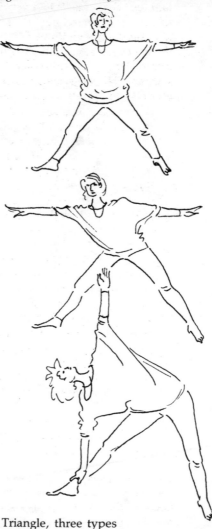

Triangle, three types

'triangle pose'. Generally, breathe out with a stretch or an effort and breathe in as you come up out of a posture.

Start off again in 'tadasana' (standing or mountain pose). Step your feet wider – 3½-4 feet apart. Inhaling, stretch your spine upwards. Exhaling stretch forwards and then bend down, hands towards the floor, back of the neck relaxed. Always bend from the tops of the thighs (where your knicker legs are!) not from the waist. Initially hold the stretch for a few seconds. Later on settle into it for longer. Notice how your lower back spreads out and stretches. Feel your hamstrings stretch. Breathing in, lift your head up. Breathing out, come all the way up.

FIGURE 1.4

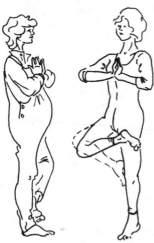

Tree, two types

Stand in 'tadasana' again. Now try this balance (Figure 1.4). Balance on your left foot and, bending your right knee, rest your right foot against your left ankle, or knee, or rest your right foot in half lotus on your left thigh. Do whichever feels right for you. Focus your eyes on something still in front of you. When you feel steady place your hands palm to palm in front of you. When that is easy, stretch your arms up above your head, palms still together. Keep breathing in a steady rhythm; keep your face and throat relaxed; don't let them tense up with effort.

This pose is called 'the tree'. Practise it balancing on your right foot too. Think of your footprint being large and broad, and energy flowing up from under the ground through your body and all your limbs.

FLOOR EXERCISES

Now come down to the floor (Figure 1.5). Keeping your back relaxed and long try these back arches. They massage and tone the abdominal organs. Make the efforts on a breath out. Hold the stretches for a few seconds at first; later, settle into them for longer. Notice how the different parts of your body feel.

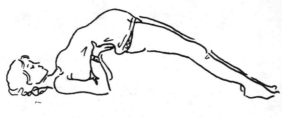

FIGURE 1.5

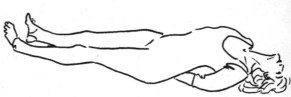

Back arches, two types

Now sit up and try the cobbler position. Bring the soles of your feet together, and release your knees down towards the floor. At first your inner thighs may feel terribly tight, but little by little the inner thighs begin to stretch and open out (Figure 1.6). Bounce your knees, butterfly-lightly, half a dozen times, then relax them downwards again. This stretch loosens the thighs and pelvic floor and stimulates the ovaries – it's invaluable. Keep your back light and lifting. Be aware of the basin of your pelvis.

FIGURE 1.6

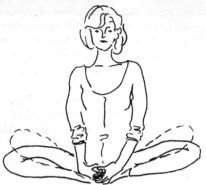

Cobbler

SHOULDER STAND AND PLOUGH

Lying down on your back bend your knees on to your chest and keep your arms by your sides. Pushing your elbows into the floor, lift your hips into the air, supporting your back with your hands. If you can, straighten your legs up into a shoulder stand. Lift up as straight as you can. After half a minute or so let your legs come down towards the floor behind *your head (put a chair behind you to rest your feet on if your legs are too tight at first).*

Notice how this strengthens your spine and abdomen, and lengthens your hamstrings (the long tendons up the backs of your legs).

Don't do these two upsidedown poses during a period because they reverse the menstrual flow. (It is unlikely, but just possible, that it could trickle back up into the fallopian tubes or even the pelvic cavity, and cause infection).

After this sequence of stretches lie down gently on your back. Starting with your feet and working up through all the muscle groups of your body, inhale, tense them a little, exhale, and release them as deeply as possible. Relax in this way from the tips of your toes to the top of your head, arms a little away from your sides, fingers lightly curled. Sink softly into the floor. Let your breathing become light

9

and undisturbed. After a little while allow your awareness to come down into your hips. Imagine the beautiful pearl white bones of your pelvis, and the rosy upsidedown pear shape of your womb, connected to the flower-like fallopian tubes that meet your ovaries. Visualize how every few weeks an egg travels down one of those tubes and floats into your womb. Allow images of fertility and plenty to fill your mind – flowers, fruits, fields of corn, anything you like that gives you a feeling of opening up and flourishing (Figure 1.7).

FIGURE 1.7

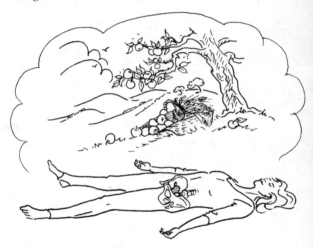

Imaginative relaxation

When you have had enough relaxation you will feel yourself 'surface' up towards the room and reality again, like a swimmer coming up from underwater. Don't leap up – wait a minute or two more, then yawn and stretch lazily like a cat. Roll over on to your left side and help yourself up with your hands.

Relaxing deeply is as vital as all the dynamic exercises. It lets you find your ability to be still, to be at peace. Like anything else, if you practise it you get better at it. Even the most frenetic of us has a peaceful side. Doing this pose (it's called 'savasana' or 'corpse pose') makes that side of ourselves more available to us.

This pre-conception session takes 15 or 20 minutes to do. None of these exercises will hurt you or the baby if you do become pregnant so don't worry about doing them in the second half of the month.

CHAPTER 2

UNFURLING LIVES: 0-3 MONTHS

You might be quite certain you are pregnant from the minute you conceive – some women know instantly. Or you might find that your pre-menstrual breast tension goes on for a few days longer than you expect and no period comes, that you have moments of feeling distinctly queasy, or suddenly tearful, for no obvious reason. This is confusing because it's so similar to the ordinary pre-menstrual sensations. However, if after a few more days (say six or seven from when the period was due) there's still no period, you could do a home pregnancy test – these cost a few pounds to buy in kit form from the chemist – but it may be worth while finding out in private whether you are or not! Do follow the instructions in the kit to the letter or you may get a false result. Most GPs ask you to wait till two weeks after your period was due before they send you to the lab with a specimen of urine. Many Women's Centres, Well Woman Clinics and all Family Planning Clinics will do a free test for you any time after you are two weeks overdue.

Then, once you have a positive test, you know it really has happened. Inside you this tiny creature is working away tremendously, growing from a tiny ball of cells into a very very small person. By the time your period is three weeks late your baby has begun to form his spine and brain – has a head and a body and tiny buds of limbs. He is about a centimetre long. By the time your period is seven weeks overdue his heart can be picked up by ultrasound. Although the movements are too delicate for you to feel, he is moving, stretching his small limbs, wriggling his body. Twelve weeks after your period was due your child has tiny arms, legs, fingers and toes, all the major organs are present in their earliest state, and his eyes are widely spaced on his broad forehead. He is then about 2½ inches long.

No wonder you feel as though there's some upheaval, something momentous going on inside you. Again, some women stay comfortable and at their ease, while many are sick, unexpectedly tired, and generally out of sorts. Just how horrible morning sickness makes you feel is generally underestimated, except by other people who've had it or are in the middle of having it. Exercise is the only remedy I've ever found for nausea. I'm not sure why it helps, but I see over and over again that it does relieve women of that symptom.

If you vomit large amounts repeatedly you may lose a lot of weight, get dehydrated, and really be quite ill. You must talk to your doctor about this and get some extra rest, perhaps even in hospital. It's sometimes a mixture of physical and emotional reaction to your pregnancy, which a few days away from your usual home situation might help. Excessive vomiting at this stage is called 'hyperemesis' or 'hyperemesis gravidarum'. After 14 or 15 weeks of pregnancy there is an excellent chance that all the queasiness will stop, of its own accord. It's as though your body gets over its surprise at the baby developing inside it.

The same thing tends to happen with the weepiness and tiredness. They usually go by the end of your third month and often don't come back until the last few weeks when you feel heavy and close to birth.

The annoying thing about this first 12 weeks is that most of the people around you don't even know you're pregnant. Nothing except larger breasts, really makes it visible. Even to you, at times, it may take an act of faith to believe this small person really exists. Because no one can see you're pregnant, you often don't get the support you could do with: you may get more help in later months, when, in actual fact, you feel far better.

Here is a stretch session, a massage and some co-counselling to use in your first 3 months. Some of the exercises were included in the 'pre-conception' exercises too. If you didn't do those read them through once now to pick up the detailed descriptions of them.

As before, what you need is loose clothing and a warm, cleared space. Sit cross-legged on the floor and steady your breathing down, lift your spine up, relax your shoulders down. Pull your bottom backwards a bit so you are sitting not on your tailbone (coccyx) but on the centre of your pelvic floor (your perineum). Notice how much more open the front of your body is if you sit this way.

Remind yourself again that you are taking a bit of time and a bit of space just for you. Use the rhythm of your breathing to think – on a breath out, breathe out tension, on a breath in, breathe in peace. When you feel you've come into the centre of yourself, stretch your neck and shoulders.

HEAD, NECK AND SHOULDERS

(These are described in detail in Chapter 1, p. 2.) Sit tall, make space in the front of your body.
1 *Drop your head forwards on to your chest, weight it with your hands. Stretch the back of your neck.*
2 *Lean your head backwards, take your upper lip up over your lower lip a few times, stretch your throat.*
3 *Lean your right ear to your right shoulder, stretch the left side of your neck.*
4 *Lean your left ear to your left shoulder, stretch the right side of your neck.*
5 *Look over your right shoulder, wait, then look a fraction further.*
6 *Look over your left shoulder, wait, then look a fraction further.*

7 *Make slow circles with your head, twice to the left, twice to the right.*

Do all this with your spine lifting, thighs, knees and ankles relaxed. Make the stretches on a breath out, lift your head up to centre on a breath in.

Now stretch your shoulders and upper chest by putting your hands palm to palm (or hold opposite elbows, or opposite wrists) behind your back, then release, slide your left arm up between your shoulder blades, reach up with your right then bend the elbow and clasp the left (or either end of a sock) (see Figure 1.2). After a few moments, change and stretch the other side.

Make all your movements as slow, strong and graceful as you can.

Now do this new stretch for your face. It is called lion pose (simhasana) and is particularly useful for relieving the fixed anxious smile long waits in the ante-natal clinic bring on. It's more fun to do with a friend as it makes you laugh. Perhaps you should organize the queue in the clinic to do it too!

Kneel back on your heels. Lift up your spine, decrease the distance between the crown of your head and the ceiling. Inhale deeply. Exhaling sharply – and do all the following at once – stretch your hands, palm down, out in front of you; curve your fingernails like claws; open your mouth as wide as possible; stick your tongue out as far as it will go; open your eyes as wide as they will go. Roar if you want to! Feel fierce! Then relax. Then do it again! (See Figure 2.1).

FIGURE 2.1

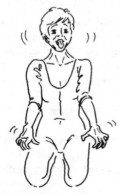

Lion pose – feels really silly at first, but it's interesting to try out being fierce

*Sit with your feet stretched out in front of you.
Alternately point and flex your feet – six points, six flexes.
Rotate your right foot at the ankle six times clockwise, six
times anticlockwise. Now do the same with your left foot.*

STANDING, BALANCING, SIDE AND FORWARD STRETCHES

*Stand in 'mountain pose' (tadasana), fully explained on p.
5, where the whole body lifts up. Make sure your hips are
rocked a little so your tailbone is tucked in. With that
movement scoop your tiny baby upwards and inwards into
your pelvis. Imagine strength flooding up through your
body through the soles of your feet. Lift the crown of your
head up to the ceiling.*

*Do 'tree pose' (vrksasana) (see p. 7), balancing first on
your left foot, right foot resting on left ankle, knee or
thigh; then balancing on your right foot. At first this is a
wobbly kind of pose, but surprisingly quickly a balance
comes. It helps to focus your eyes on something – put on a
table in front of you a flower, a favourite stone or shell, or
if you are exercising in the evening, light a candle. One of
my students always did all her stretching by candlelight.
She didn't care how bizarre her family thought it was, she
knew intuitively that the soft half-light was just right for
finding the instinctive, sensual rhythms of birth. When
her baby came, she was born in candlelight too.*

*Now take your feet 3-3½ feet apart and do the side
stretch 'trikonasana' or 'triangle pose', described on p. 6.
Never forget to check that when you work to the right, the
right heel is in line with the left instep, and when you
work to the left, vice versa. When you work to the right
make space along the right-hand side of the body; don't
collapse or crumple it. When you work to the left, make
space on the left side of your body.*

*Make all your movements as strong, slow and graceful
as you can. Always try to keep your face and throat
relaxed. Now step your feet wide apart, 4-4½ feet – feet
parallel and toes pointing forwards. Breathing in, stretch
forwards; breathing out, release down, bending at the top*

of the thighs, not the back of the waist (see p. 7). When your legs feel strong and confident in this pose you can put your hands palm to palm (or hold opposite wrists, or opposite elbows) behind your back when you do it. Breathing in, lift your head up then breathing out, bring your torso up all in one movement (don't 'uncurl' up). Keep your back broad and flat throughout this and any other forward stretch.

Bring your feet together and turn your right foot out at an angle of 45°. Step your left foot forwards about 3 feet. Put your hands on your hips. Breathe in, lift up your spine. Breathing out, stretch your upper body forwards, and when you reach your comfortable maximum for the day, bend downwards. Experience the stretch in the backs of your legs and your lower back. As with the other poses, a few seconds of this stretch (it's called 'parsvottanasana') each side will be quite enough at first. Later on you will settle into it for longer, and will want to put your hands palm to palm behind your back (Figure 2.2). Keep

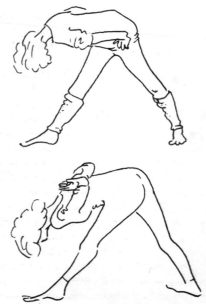

FIGURE 2.2

Standing forward bend, two types

breathing steadily – don't concentrate so hard on stretching that you forget to breathe! To come up, breathe in and lift your head up, and breathing out, lift the rest of your torso up all in one piece. Don't 'uncurl' up.

All these standing stretches strengthen your legs and make them more supple. This helps to carry the increasing weight of your baby over the months and, as you will see later, is also very important in helping you to keep moving during labour.

Stand with your feet about 3 feet apart. Lift your spine and release your shoulders. Put your hands together in front of your chest. Knees are straight. Keep your hips still and move your ribs to the right (slowly), centre them, then to the left, then centre them. If you're not sure what's going on try it out in front of a mirror, or get a friend to hold your hips still while you get the upper part of your body to move on its own! Stretch left-centre-right-centre slowly, noticing what stretches where, half a dozen times. Don't have your legs and hips tense, just firm and still (Figure 2.3).

FIGURE 2.3

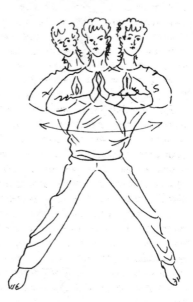

Rib isolations – don't twist, just *slide* across

Then put your hands on your hips and bend your knees slightly. Really slowly, rock your hips backwards and forwards in a big arc. Feel what moves in your back, thighs and pelvis floor. Do it really slowly half-a-dozen times. Straighten your knees up and let your legs rest a bit. Bend your knees slightly again and lift your hips up to the right as far as you can (come on to your tiptoes with your right foot) then down to centre, then up to your left. Again, see what happens in your back, thighs and pelvic floor. Straighten up, rest your knees. Bend them slightly again and make very big, very slow circles with your hips – six to the right, then six to the left. Straighten your legs. Now sit down for your floor exercises.

FLOOR EXERCISES

Sit tall. I keep saying sit or stand tall because these exercises are only about a tenth as effective if you do them with a collapsed, compacted spine. Inside your spine is your spinal cord. This cord carries your central nervous system. Your central nervous system handles some tremendously strong sensations during birth. It is useful to have a strong and supple spine which you can keep moving around and stretching in different ways, rather than one which flops about and can't do anything for itself.

So, with that lecture over, sit tall! Stretch your legs out as wide as you can to the sides and put the backs of your palms on the fronts of your knees. If you're doing your yoga with a friend you can extend each other's stretch – carefully – by sitting foot to foot. Make sure (Figure 2.4) you are still sitting on your perineum, not your tailbone – that is, on the middle of your pelvic floor, not on the back of it. It may mean you have to bring your legs in a little closer together, but it's better to do that and have a free back. Imagine your spine. Now imagine the front of your spine, which faces your tummy, your lungs, etc. Always try to stretch the front of your spine as well as the back of it and your body will begin to loosen up all over and move much better.

Still sitting with your legs stretched wide apart, breathe

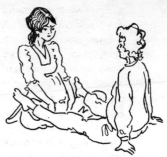

FIGURE 2.4

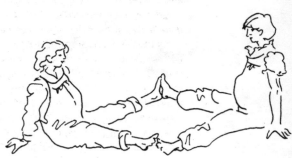

Pair sole to sole, and pair feet on opposite knees

in and stretch your spine upwards. Breathing out, walk your hands forward between your legs and stretch your whole body forwards. The stretch is in the hip joints and the lower back, not the back of the waist. It's better to go 2 inches forward with a broad, free back than 2 feet forwards hunched up and constricting your tummy. In time you will lie on the floor – although unless you're already supple your baby is going to get there first as you will be making this stretch over a bigger and bigger bump. So do what is right for you on each particular day. All that matters is that you loosen in the hips and the back, with a strong and easy stretch, not that you strain yourself to 'achieve' some 'ideal position'.

Friends working foot-to-foot together can pull one another gently forwards alternatively, like in the children's 'row your boat' game. Be sensitive to your partner. You will feel when she comes to the tight place in her stretch, don't pull her further than she is ready to go.

Now your thighs are well warmed up and loosened. Bring your feet together sole to sole, hold your feet and flop your knees with gentle little flops towards the floor. Be careful to keep your spine flying up out of the floor even if it makes your knees come up a bit. Breathe down towards your hip joints. See if you can let go a little more. Stay as long as you comfortably can.

Friends working together can gently weight each other's knees towards the floor, as in Figure 2.4.

After making this stretch, lift your knees up gently with your hands and stretch your legs out in front of you.

As well as increasing the stretches by working in pairs, you can do all of your floor exercises back to back if you are tired, or miserable, or just very fond of the person you're working with. There is something very comforting and pleasant about the warmth and strength of somebody else's spine leaning against yours. If you decide to work in this way, keep wriggling your hips close together – keep your lower backs touching as well as your shoulders.

Having opened your hips outwards let's now turn the thighs the other way. Kneel up, separate your feet behind you, and then carefully lower yourself down so that you're sitting between your feet. If your knees feel very tight, don't stay; use your hands to lift yourself up and arrange some cushions between your feet and try again. If that still feels bad, take the cushions away, and try with one leg stretched in front of you and one bent round to the side. Separate your knees if you need to but be working to bring them together. This is called 'virasana' or 'hero pose' (see Figure 2.5). Make yourself tall, and keep both the front and the back of your body open. Clasp your hands and breathe in. Breathing out, turn your palms away from you and stretch them out in front of you then right up above your head – palms facing the ceiling. Send energy from the palms of your hands up to the ceiling. Breathe steadily. Notice how your shoulders and upper arms are working. Breathe out and float your arms away from you and downwards. If you have one leg forward, change legs. Clasp your hands again, this time with the other index

FIGURE 2.5

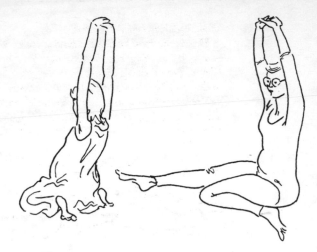

Virasana, two types

*finger on top. It feels as though you have an extra finger!
Now on a breath out stretch upwards again, palms to the
ceiling. When you get used to this pose, make the stretch
up come from the floor, not just from your armpits. Hold
the upward stretch for 5 or 10 seconds, longer if it's
comfortable. Don't hold your breath. On a breath out, float
your arms outwards and downwards. If you are supple
you can lie back in hero pose, taking your weight first
on your elbows, then on the crown of your head, then
sliding on to your back. If you aren't as loose as this, try,
carefully, lying back on a large pile of cushions or beanbag.*

*Come up on to all fours. Breathe in. On the breath out
arch your back, slowly and gracefully like a cat. On the
breath in flatten it (don't dip it in the centre). Breathing
out, arch; breathing in flatten, slowly, six more times.
Settle on to all fours again. Breathe in; on the breath out
look round at your right hip. Move the hip towards your
head a little. Breathe in, come to the centre. Breathing out,
look to your left hip; move your left hip towards your head
a little. Slowly, in the rhythm of your breathing, do it six
more times each way. Then bring your feet together, move
your knees wider apart, and on a breath out stretch your
bottom towards your feet and your chest towards the floor.*

This stretch is called frog pose.

This is the most important stretch we've tried so far and you will probably use it a tremendous amount during labour. Don't worry if you don't get your upper body on to the floor, get a pile of cushions or pillows, or a beanbag, and resting your bottom on your heels, make yourself as long as you can and lie forwards on your support (see Figure 2.6).

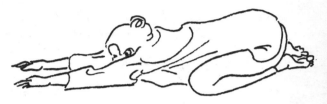

FIGURE 2.6

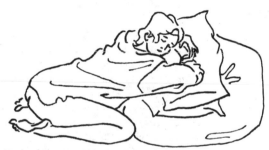

Frog pose, two types

In this position your pelvis is wide open, your lower back and tailbone free to stretch, and your hips are mobile. We will be using it over and over again.

Stay in this stretch a little longer each time you try it. To come up, breathe in, lift your head, press your hands into the floor. Breathing out, walk your hands back and lift yourself up.

SHOULDER STAND AND PLOUGH

Once you know you are pregnant, unless you have been doing inverted positions for years, it is better to drop doing them. They will not hurt you or your baby for the first couple of weeks until you get your pregnancy test results, but it is better to leave them after that unless you are very experienced.

If you are experienced and you do want to carry on, do keep getting your yoga teacher to have a look at you in the inverted posture, and make sure that everything is alright. She or he will be able to tell from things like the colour of your face and the tension or relaxation of the muscles in your neck, whether it is wise for you to continue.

RELAXATION

Sometimes it's pleasant to listen to slow, peaceful music during relaxation. Sometimes silence (if that's available in your house!) is more relaxing. In the daytime try drawing the curtains to make it darker; at night lower the lights. Lie yourself down on your back. Lift your head and see if the centre line of your body is straight. If not, straighten it. Lower your head on to the floor. Now, breathing steadily, begin to tighten a bit, then relax deeply, each group of muscles. Tighten slightly on a breath in, let go completely on a breath out. Do this with your feet, knees and calves, hips, shoulders, hands and arms, face and throat. Then you are relaxed from the tips of your toes to the top of your head. Sink heavily and warmly into the floor. Imagine a place where you would like to be – a tropical beach, a sunny hillside, anywhere, real or imagined, where you feel at peace. Imagine you are there. Your breathing will be light and gentle. After a few minutes for yourself alone, without disturbing yourself, move your hand on to your lower abdomen, very low down. Under your hand your baby is growing. Say hello to your baby, say anything you want to say to her, just silently in your own mind.

Here are some of the things mothers have told me they've said to their very young babies:

'Hello. Who are you?' 'You were a bit of a surprise!' 'Are you allright in there?' 'You're making me feel rotten, but I'm glad you're there.' 'I'm afraid of you

*and what you're going to mean to my life.' 'I wish I
could feel you more, or see my tummy getting bigger.'*

*When you've had enough relaxation, you will feel
yourself begin to drift back to reality, back into the room.
Blink your eyes open. Stretch your fingers, stretch your
toes. Stretch your arms and legs. Roll over on to your left
side and curl up there for a minute or two. Then, pressing
your hands into the floor, help yourself up to a sitting
position. Don't rush around. Give yourself a few more
minutes to tune into life again.*

CO-COUNSELLING

Co-counselling is a simple way in which friends or
partners can give each other a chance to talk about
the things which are important to them. With a
friend who is expecting a baby too, you could use
the same topics. With a male partner you could use
these topics and he could explore his thoughts about
being a father. A female partner too needs time to
work out what the coming baby means to her. With
other friends you could give them some time on
other issues.

Co-counselling is not a discussion, it is an
exchange of really good listening on one side and a
chance to talk quite freely without any interruption
at all on the other. The talker should let herself say
absolutely anything she wants for her (agreed
beforehand) time – say 5 or 10 minutes. The listener
should sit opposite, both of you comfortable, and
the listener should keep eye contact and be attentive
all the time, but not say anything at all, until the 5 or
10 minutes are over. It sounds, and is, quite simple,
but it's surprising how much more you find out
about what you think and feel if you have time and
'permission' to talk. Afterwards, of course, you can
share reactions to what you said, but for the actual
counselling part of it you should have time entirely
for yourself to talk. Then you change around and
the listener talks, while the talker listens. This is

much more balanced then the classical 'therapy' situation where the listener never talks and gets more and more powerful because they know more and more about the talker's inner life and never share any of their own. You may feel very self-conscious when you first try this out, but surprisingly quickly it comes to feel an ordinary and sensible kind of thing to do.

When you first become pregnant many things may be worth co-counselling about. For example:

how you feel about being pregnant;
how you feel about being a mother in the future;
how you feel about sharing your body with another (albeit small) person;
anything else which is important to you at this time.

MASSAGE

Living in a woman's body in this society is never going to be easy. Bombarded by advertising and pornography which suggests (a) that only certain shapes of body are beautiful and (b) that women's bodies are only consumer items for the use of men; knowing that advertising and pornography express the deeply ingrained attitudes of this society, we are all vulnerable all the time. Pregnancy makes it even more difficult and complicated. If you're a pregnant woman, what happens to your sexuality (in other people's eyes, even if it doesn't change in your own)? What happens to your status at work if you work outside the home? If you work at home do you feel even more labelled 'housewife', 'mother', 'cabbage'? Because you have probably had to fight for whatever identity and visual image you have already formed for yourself, it is particularly hard to have that image changing with your changing shape. As you climb, for example, out of black leathers into a floral smock, the shock is hard to handle!

That is why the massage for the first 3 months is a

facial massage. Much of our identity is expressed in our features. It is useful to soothe and relax them at this time.

Face massage

If you are the one being massaged lie on your back and relax. Your only task is to say if the massager is stroking you too firmly. If you are the massager, kneel with a knee each side of your friend's face (see Figure 2.7). Calm yourself down; make sure you are not going to transmit tension or anxiety through your hands.

FIGURE 2.7

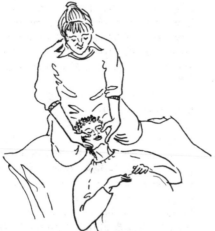

Face massage, pairs

First of all make lots of slow smooth light strokes with the whole of your hands from your partner's chin to the crown of her head. If she has long hair, scoop her hair up behind her from under her neck. Get the feel of the shape of her skull.

Then, with one thumb, gently begin to stroke up and down a vertical line in the centre of her brow. This releases a tremendous amount of tension in the brow. Notice what you can feel with your thumb. When you feel a 'letting-go' in the forehead, rest your hands on either side of your partner's brow.

Starting at the top of the forehead and working down to the eyebrows, make firm but gentle strokes with both thumbs from the centre lines outwards. When you get down to the eyebrows, using the fingertips make small circles at the temples. Make half-a-dozen in one direction, and half-a-dozen in the other. By now your partner is probably very still, breathing lightly, and with a blissful expression! Now rest your hands on either side of her face. Again make strokes with your thumbs, gently under the brows but over the eyes, then along the lower edge of the eye sockets, then from the bridge of the nose outwards. Work down the whole face, including the upper lip and the chin. Then reach your hands down under her neck and with your index and middle fingers stroke gently the length of the back of the neck several times. Lastly lift her head gently from underneath with both hands, stretch her neck, tucking her chin in, very, very gently. Give her a few minutes to come round! Then change places.

When you are doing the massage, notice what you feel through your hands, and how much calm you can induce with them. When your baby is born much of your communication with her will be by touch, as will hers with you. It's useful to have become more sensitive to touch and feeling during pregnancy.

When you are being massaged, you may find this particular massage releases a few tears. Let them come, they are a 'letting-go' too. In this position they will trickle into your ears!

CHAPTER 3

AN EASY-GOING PARTNERSHIP: 3-6 MONTHS

These are often a good 3 months. With any luck, the sickness and peculiar tiredness goes, and the movements made by the growing baby are felt by you. First, at 16 or 17 weeks, a flutter which might or might not be, then a little kick which almost certainly is, then a great wriggle, and you know someone in there is choosing to move when she wants, and strongly enough for you to feel it. It's somehow much easier to know the baby as a person in her own right once you can feel her choosing when to move and when to sleep. Before long it's not so much a delicate fluttering as a feeling as though you had a little sea-lion inside you, diving and tumbling in the bag of waters. She can also suck her thumb, drink sips of amniotic fluid, and pass urine (don't worry, the amniotic fluid is renewed every few hours, and her waste products are carried off to be dealt with by your kidneys). She can hear sounds and music, she knows whether it's light or dark, she knows whether you are still or moving. If you sunbathe (in moderation only) with a bare tummy, her world changes from a deep, dusky purple environment to a redcurrant red one, as your abdomen wall thins when your womb stretches, and more light can come in.

With a first baby, by 16 or 17 weeks and often earlier with second and subsequent babies, as a uterus that has expanded once seems to expand more quickly the next time, a distinct bump begins to show. Very tight trousers will have been uncomfortable for a long time, because the increase in fluid retention will have made you a little fuller over your tummy anyway, but after 16 weeks it's not unusual to find you can't do up your ordinary skirts and trousers. Whether you can buy maternity clothes that express your personality without costing a fortune depends a bit on what fashion in general is doing. During a phase where loose, flowing and voluminous clothes are in favour it is easy to find accommodating clothes which aren't specialist 'maternity' or specialist prices. This has the added advantage that you don't feel too conspicuous too soon. When street fashion dictates tight, clinging or restricting styles, it's harder to find anything interesting and reasonably priced to wear.

Pregnancy is a time when some women simply want to economize on clothes and look forward to getting back into their ordinary things; some women love their swelling curves and dress to emphasize them; some want to conceal their pregnancy as long as possible; and for some it's a positive breaking of bounds – at last, exactly because of their changing shape, they can stop bothering to aim for a man-made image of femalekind and find their own way of looking. Finding a personal style doesn't have to be expensive and the confidence it gives lasts after your baby is born. Trust your own feelings; do what suits you. However, if you find yourself identifying with each of those states described above in turn, and therefore feeling pretty confused, try doing some co-counselling on the subject (see the end of this chapter).

To exercise, a really stretchy leotard which wasn't too tight in the first place will last right through your pregnancy (but it will never be the same again!). Always exercise in bare feet or footless tights; it's safer and allows your feet and toes to spread and develop while you work. Legwarmers are useful over ankles and calves in cold weather, but don't pull them down over your heels as illustrated in some books – you'll fall over them. If you choose a tracksuit make sure the waist will pull well up over your bump, i.e. make sure it is quite long in the body. Cotton jumpsuits or boilersuits and loose dungarees look as though they would be alright, but non-stretchy material will cut into your thighs and other places while you do your exercises, – so in fact a loose dress is better than any of these. In summer a bathing suit or bikini is fine. Probably best of all would be to wear nothing at all working in a warm, softly lit, quiet room with a soft, clean carpet (Figure 3.1). Chance would be a fine thing (but maybe you *can* arrange to do this).

FIGURE 3.1

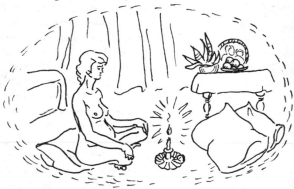

Nude, by candlelight

STRETCH SESSION

The stretch session for this 3 months concentrates on strengthening and stretching your lower back muscles which carry much of the weight as the size of your baby increases to the front. We also keep loosening and working on the neck and shoulder muscles to keep your balance and posture, and keep your abdominals active without overstressing them. We go on loosening the thighs, and begin to activate and strengthen the pelvic floor. It's important now because the heavy uterus is pressing down on this sling of muscles and later, during birth, you will want to know how to relax and stretch them. After your baby is born you will want to tone the muscles up again so they can return to their usual strength. The session also includes some breathing exercises. If you haven't done the pre-conception exercises, and those for 0-3 months, read them through now, because some of them are used again in this session. Then read this session through once, slowly, and practise it for the first few times with the book next to you. The sequence of stretches will soon become easy to remember, or you could, as suggested before, make yourself a tape of instructions.

CENTRING YOURSELF

Sit cross-legged on the floor. Pull your buttocks back a little way to make sure you are sitting on the centre of your pelvic floor. Sit on the points of your buttock bones rather than your tailbone (your coccyx). By doing this and by lifting your spine up and releasing your shoulders down, notice how much more space you are making in the front of your body. Now the baby is growing you can feel how important this is. Let the crown of your head lift up towards the ceiling. Now close your eyes and let your breathing become a little deeper than usual. Hear your breath coming and going. Keeping your spine light and lifting, collect up in your mind any distractions and worries, and begin to breathe them away. Remind yourself that this is your time, that the next half an hour is just for you. Begin to think − on the breath out, breathe out tension, on the breath in, breathe in peace. Continue to centre yourself in this way, breathing away tension, inhaling a sense of calm and peace, until you feel centred and focused on yourself. Your baby may well join in by dancing about with delight. This is because slow, steady breathing may increase her oxygen supply − your extra well-oxygenated blood flowing through to her through your placenta.

If you ever get dizzy doing this, or any other special breathing, stop at once and let your breathing return to normal. It isn't likely to happen, but it's good to be aware that you shouldn't just go on if it does. Cup your hands over your face and breathe a few breaths like that. Pause and rest for a few minutes, then try breathing out again with a little less emphasis. If it still happens, don't do special breathing at all; you can still use the idea 'breathe in peace, breathe out tension' with a quite everyday level of breath.

When you feel ready, rub your hands together to warm them, cup your face in your warm hands, and blink your eyes open behind your hands. When your eyes are used to the light, float your hands down into your lap.

Now stretch your head, neck and shoulders (described in detail on p. 2).

1 Sit tall. Breathing out, drop your head forwards on to your chest; weight it with your clasped hands. Feel the stretch in the back of your neck. Breathe steadily.
2 Breathe in, lift your head up; breathe out, drop it back. Take your upper lip up over your lower lip a few times; stretch your throat. Keep your spine lifting; keep breathing steadily.
3 Breathe in, lift your head up; breathing out, drop your right ear to your right shoulder; stretch the left side of your neck.
4 Breathe in, lift up; breathe out, drop your right ear to your right shoulder; stretch the left side of your neck.
5 Breathe in, lift your head up. Breathe out, look round over your right shoulder. Stay there and breathe in. Breathing out, look a fraction further. Breathing in, come back to centre.
6 Breathe out, look over your left shoulder. Stay there and breathe in. Breathing out, look a fraction further. Breathe in and come back to centre.

Make sure you're still sitting up with the back and the front of your spine (try to visualize it) stretching upwards, and with your shoulders relaxing down.

Make slow circles with your whole head, twice to the left, twice to the right.

Now place the back of your left hand on the outside of your right knee. Breathing in, stretch out and then behind you with your right arm, place your right hand on the floor behind you. Look over your right shoulder (Figure

FIGURE 3.2

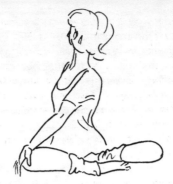

Sitting twist – feel a stretch but not a strain

3.2). *Keep your face and throat relaxed and keep breathing steadily. When you first learn this twist hold it for 5 or 10 seconds. After a while you will be able to hold it comfortably for 20-30 seconds. Feel a stretch, but not a strain. Remind yourself that yoga is an exploration, not a competition.*

When you've had enough, on a breath out, release and face the front.

Now twist the other way. Raise your spine, put the back of your right hand on the outside of your left knee. On a breath out stretch your left arm out to the side, then behind you; place your left hand on the floor behind you. Look back over your left shoulder. Notice how this is gently toning your abdominal muscles, especially the long ones which make diagonals from centre ribs to outside hips, and is moving the back of your waist.

Now, stand up slowly.

STANDING, ARM STRENGTHENING

Stand in 'mountain pose' or 'tadasana' (described in detail on p. 5). Make sure your weight is evenly distributed between left and right foot, between the heels and the balls of your feet. Rise up strong and tall from these strong, even footprints. Be particularly careful to adjust your hips so that your tailbone is tucked in. Feel how this takes pressure off the sling of muscles across the lowest part of your abdomen, because by scooping your baby backwards and upwards in this way, you take some of the weight off that part of your tummy. Remember to release your shoulders backwards and downwards and to let your head lift at the crown. Take your gaze to the floor 2 or 3 yards ahead of you and breathe steadily. Relax your eyes by thinking of an animal that has gentle eyes and and getting some of that gentle feeling in your own eyes. Remain for a minute or more in this pose.

If you have been using this book for several weeks already, 'mountain pose' will be coming naturally to you. Keep exploring how you can make more and more space in your body as you do it. Always do mountain pose (without gazing at the floor!) in queues, on escalators, anywhere you have to stand for a long time. It's surprisingly revitalizing.

Now stepping your feet 2 or 3 feet apart, learn three arm strengthening exercises. When your baby is born you will be pleased to have strengthened your arms as you carry your child around, hold her close to feed or cuddle, not to mention lifting so called carrycots all over the place (the last thing they're any use for is carrying) and dealing with bulky packs of nappies and bundles of laundry (Figure 3.3).

FIGURE 3.3

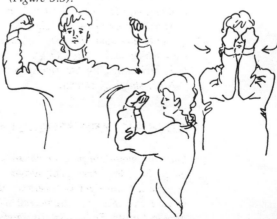

Hands across chest then flung out

35

Arms stretched out to the sides, palms up, make gentle fists. On a breath out bend your arms up at the elbows. Now bring your elbows together in front of you, take them out to the sides, together, apart together, apart, rhythmically. Start with eight repetitions and build up day by day till you can do twenty-four.

Secondly Figure 3.4 bring your arms out to the sides, shoulder level. Cross your hands across your chest once, twice, then fling your arms back at shoulder level. Look behind you before you start, it's excruciating to collide with the wall! Do this eight times at first, and gradually build up to twenty-four.

FIGURE 3.4

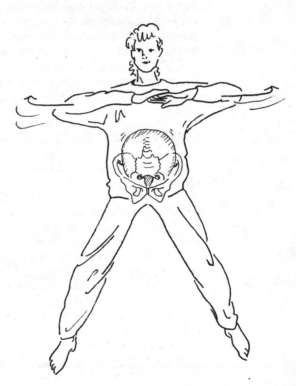

Bent arms brought forward, three types

Thirdly, stand 18 inches to 2 feet away from the wall, feet a little apart and pointing straight forward. Place your hands, fingers pointing inwards, on the wall. Breathe in, and keeping your body straight, bend your elbows out to the sides, and lean into the wall. Breathing out, press on your palms and straighten your arms, pushing yourself upright again, keeping your body straight. These are wall press-ups. Start with eight and work up day by day until you can do twenty-four.

After your three arm-strengthening exercises, shake your arms out well.

Incidentally, having strong arms has other implications for women, quite apart from being comfortable carrying their babies. With our arms we hold on to what we want, and push away what we don't want: it's appropriate that a feeling of personal power increases if our arms are stronger. Making your arms stronger will mean that any self-defence or martial arts training you might choose to do at some other time will come more easily to you, and you will be able to use it with more power.

FORWARD AND SIDE BENDING

Find a sturdy piece of furniture, table height. A heavy table that won't slip, kitchen units, etc. are ideal. Stand a couple of feet away from it in tadasana (see p. 5). Hold the edge. Breathe in and stretch your spine upwards; breathing out, bend at the tops of the thighs, not in the waist, and slowly walk backwards until your legs are vertical and your torso horizontal, parallel with the floor. Let your spine sink deep into your body; make your back as flat and broad as possible. Stay there breathing steadily and experience the stretch in your hamstrings and imagine the triangle of your lower back spreading out. After a few seconds breathe in and lift your head up; breathing out, walk towards the table and stand up. Then do the whole thing again. If you are working with a friend she can feel all over your back and show you where the tense parts are (anywhere that humps upwards, or with ridges of spine sticking up). She can gently but firmly massage those parts with circles of the fingertips or the heel of her hand. Then change over, and you feel for the tight parts of her back, and see if you can soothe them out a little.

This simple stretch is effective for getting rid of pregnancy backaches. In many cases, after a few days of stretching in this way, the ache goes altogether.

As with all the other exercises, hold it for just a few seconds at first, but for a little longer each day.

Now stand up again and stretch to the side (trikonasana or triangle pose, explained on p. 5). Work both the left and the right side.

Come up again, and stepping one foot forward, stretch to the front (parsvothanasana, explained on p. 17).

Balancing first on one foot, then on the other, do tree pose (p. 7). Feel how this brings strength to your thighs.

FIGURE 3.5

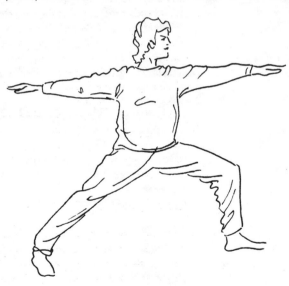

Warrior pose – powerful women

Now learn one more standing pose, which also strengthens your legs. It is called warrior pose 2, or virabhadrasana 2 (see Figure 3.5). (Virabhadrasana 1 and 3 are not suitable for pregnancy.) Step your feet 4-4½ feet apart, and turn your left foot in, right foot out. Breathe in, bring your arms out to shoulder level; breathe out, release your shoulders and extend your fingertips. Breathe in again, and on the breath out bend the right knee so the shin is vertical and the thigh horizontal. Look along to your right middle fingertip. Keep your spine vertical and your body open and facing the front. Stay only for a few seconds at first. Breathe in, straighten your knee and come up and, breathing out, release your arms down. Then repeat to the other side. Ideally you need a friend to check this pose for you, or do it in front of a mirror so you can see whether you are doing it correctly. The most common mistake is to bend the bent knee so far that it goes beyond the foot – don't do this – stretch and lower the thigh more, and keep the knee just above the foot, the shin vertical.

After warrior pose practise rib isolations (see p. 18) and then hip circles. Soon the distance you can extend in both these will increase a great deal. Make eight stretches each way with your ribs, then eight circles each way with your hips (knees slightly bent for this), and eight large rocking movements forwards and backwards with your hips.

All these movements should be slow, strong and sensual. If you move sharply you risk pulling muscles – long muscles on your abdomen, or muscles in your lower back. Making the movements part of a dance to some music that makes you feel uninhibited is a good way of practising them.

ON ALL FOURS

Now come down on to all fours. Space your hands and feet evenly; distribute the weight evenly between them. To the slow rhythm of your own steady breathing, arch and flatten your back – arching on a breath out, flattening on a breath in. Repeat this a dozen or so times. Your arms, wrists and thighs are strengthened, your spine extended.

Separate your knees wider and put your feet together. On a breath out stretch your bottom back towards your feet and your chest and face to the ground. Rest forward on to pillows or a big beanbag if the stretch is too much for you at first. Let go in the lower back.

FIGURE 3.6

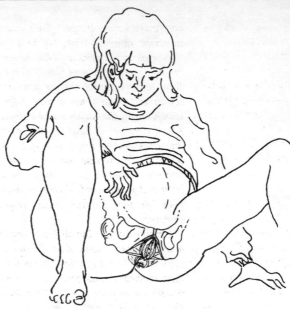

Pelvic floor muscles

In this position exercise your pelvic floor. Imagine you are dying to go to the toilet but there is nowhere near at hand where you could. Tighten the muscles you would tighten in that situation – those are your pelvic floor muscles (see Figure 3.6). Then let them go. Contract, release, contract, release, then on a breath in lift your head up, on a breath out, walk your hands back to your body to help yourself up. At first this may be very awkward and frustrating if you haven't been aware of those muscles before. Or you may recognize these as the muscles that pulse involuntarily when you have an orgasm. Anyhow, with practice you can contract and release them at will, and even contract or release the vagina or the back passage separately if you want to. As your baby grows the heavy womb puts pressure on these muscles – it is necessary to make them stronger. When you become familiar with and confident about this part of you, it's far easier to contemplate opening wide enough to allow your baby to slide through as she's born. After your baby's born it is these exercises which bring your vagina back to its familiar size and shape. If you don't choose to do any other exercises from this book, try to do pelvic floor squeezes!

A good way we have found to make these part of life is to buy some sticky paper stars. Take five of these and stick them around your house or flat in places where you will see them several times a day – for example, one by the kettle, one in the corner of the bathroom mirror, and so on. Every time you see a star you do ten pelvic floor squeeze-and-releases – ending with a gentle squeeze. This way you perform the exercise many, many times a day, but it's never a nuisance. Leave the stars up at least until your baby is 3 months old. Carry on doing them for the rest of your life; they improve sexual response and help prevent prolapse.

Coming back to the all fours sequence, resting on hands and knees make some slow, sexy circles with your hips – eight times one way, eight times the other. Now rock your hips backwards and forwards, so your weight goes first, mostly on to your wrists, then mostly on to your knees. Do this eight times.

Separate your knees and put your feet together; stretch down to the floor (or your cushions) again. Squeeze and release your pelvic floor another eight times, finishing with a gentle squeeze.

Get up from this stretch slowly then sit up.

SITTING SEQUENCE – LOOSENING AND STRETCHING THE THIGHS

1 Sit tall. Stretch your legs as wide apart as possible. Push your heels away. Rest the backs of your hands on the fronts of your knees (explained in detail on p. 19).
2 On a breath out walk your hands forward, stretching your straight spine downwards. Don't arch your back to get your head lower. It's a far more useful loosening to go a couple of inches forwards with the front of your spine open than to hunch down bending at the waist. This will only hurt your back (explained in detail on p. 20).
3 Put the soles of your feet together bring your heels as close in to your body as you can. Release your knees down

towards the floor. If you have been practising these exercises for several weeks you will notice that your thighs are already opening quite a bit wider. Gloat for a moment over the fact that the changing hormones of pregnancy mean that any work you do on becoming supple is effective much more quickly than for someone doing the same amount of work who isn't pregnant. Always keep your body lifting up from your base on the floor. Those of you who have followed the book for some weeks will be finding this lifting posture coming much more naturally now.

4 Stretch your thighs the other way by putting your knees together, and feet apart, and sitting down between your feet. Place cushions between your feet if your knees are tight. (See detailed explanation on p. 21). Stretch your arms up above your head.

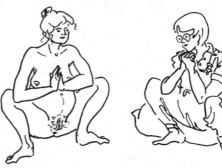

FIGURE 3.7

Squat, two types

5 Start to become used to a squatting position (Figure 3.7). At first use your hands to support you and let your heels come up off the floor, but work to get your heels on the floor and, eventually, also to put your hands together and press your knees a little further apart. Straighten first one leg, then bend it and straighten the other, pushing the heel away, to stretch your thighs a little more (Figure 3.8).

Squat as often as you can. You are stretching your thighs and your perineum, opening your pelvis to its widest, and becoming familiar with one of the most useful positions for labour and birth. When your baby is sitting

FIGURE 3.8

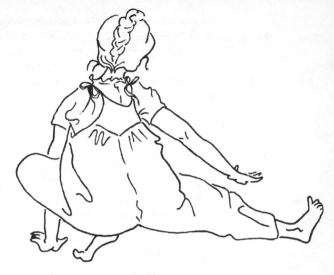

Squat, one leg extended

up and crawling you will mostly want to play with her on the floor and will be far more comfortable if you can squat easily. When you first start to feed her solids she will be happier in a 'bouncy chair' than wobbling around in a high chair, and again, an easy squat is the most comfortable position for you to settle into to spoonfeed her.

Constipation, which can be a nuisance during pregnancy, is eased both by practising squatting and by squatting on the loo seat (hold on to something stable!) if you're having trouble.

Piles, another irritation of pregnancy, can be eased by a combination of practising pelvic floor squeezes, practising squatting (keeping circulation and muscle tone good in the anal sphincter) and eating plenty of bran, fruit and vegetables to keep the contents of your bowels soft. It's well worth it – a sore bottom can feel like the last straw during pregnancy, and repeated painful bowel movements lessen your confidence about pushing your baby out easily through your vagina.

After practising squatting rest your legs for a moment. Then cross your legs and sit up. If you are tired by now sit back to back with a friend, or sit with your back supported by cushions, a beanbag, the front of an armchair, or anything comfortable. Now it is time to start to concentrate on breathing.

BREATHING\AWARENESS

If you have been following the exercises in this book, you will already have become used to making stretches, efforts, etc. on a breath out. *This is the most useful breathing awareness of all, and you can use it during labour, birth, and then any other strenuous or creative movement – dance, self-defence, yoga, not to mention everyday lifting and pushing and manoeuvring.*

Here is a special way of breathing which will carry you through your baby's birth.

Place one hand on your lower abdomen, below your navel. Close your eyes.

1 *Breathe in a steady rhythm, a little more slowly than usual.*
2 *Once your rhythm is established start to breathe in through your nose and out through your mouth. Don't blow, let the air escape out through your mouth.*
3 *When that is coming easily take your awareness down to the hand on your tummy. Direct the breath in all the way down to the hand so that your tummy expands and pushes your hand out a little. Make the breath out come all the way up from behind your hand, so that your tummy collapses back away from your hand a little.*
4 *Continue this deep breathing, for a minute or two at first – gradually build up to 4 or 5 minutes every day. Notice how still and calm you become. A classroom full of people doing this breathing comes quiet and full of peace.*

RELAXATION

When you've had enough breathing, without disturbing yourself at all, lie down to do relaxation. Relax lying on your left side, one pillow under your head, and another under your right knee. Once you get past about 24 weeks this is better than lying on your back, which might give you backache, and also makes your heavy womb squash some of the major blood vessels.

Don't miss out on relaxation. Squeeze, then on a breath out, let go all the muscle groups from your toes to your head (described in detail on p. 10). Take yourself in your imagination to your favourite landscape – a warm seashore, a sunny garden, wherever you like. After a while, gently put your hand on to your abdomen and have a chat with your child. At this time in the pregnancy the baby will often swim up to meet your hand and push his hands or feet against your hand.

When you feel yourself floating back up to the surface again, you have finished your relaxation. Don't jump up and start rushing around – yawn and stretch for a while first, then press your hands into the floor and help yourself up that way.

CO-COUNSELLING

With a friend or partner spend a few moments making a list of the topics you want to talk about. These might include feelings about giving up work, dealing with other people's reactions to your coming baby, and anything else that feels important now. Many women dream vividly throughout pregnancy, especially once they can feel the baby move. If a vivid dream or nightmare has stayed in your mind try describing it. Without trying to 'analyse' it too much see if the message or feelings contained in the dream arise in your mind more clearly as you speak.

Co-counsel, as described in Chapter 2, for an agreed length of time and see what develops or clarifies itself. Afterwards, share your reactions to each other's thoughts.

MASSAGE

The person to be massaged should start by sitting cross-legged. The person doing the massaging should start by taking a few calming breaths herself or himself and making sure he or she is not bringing tension to her friend in her hands. To make sure you do not impose your ego or worries on anyone you want to massage, it can help to say to yourself silently as you take some deep breaths 'my hands are empty – my heart is open'.

Now stroke your friend's neck for a few seconds, then gently begin to knead her shoulders with your fingertips and thumbs. When the shoulders begin to feel soft and loose work your way down her spine, massaging with whatever sort of stroking feels pleasant to both of you, from the spine out to the sides of the body. Try small circles with your fingertips, or smooth stroking movements with the whole hand. Go all the way down the spine, in a leisurely fashion, two or three times. Now ask her to lie down gently on her side.

Make big, strong circles with the heel of your hand, starting in the centre of the lower back, and coming round over the hip (Figure 3.9). Loosen the whole hip. Many women describe feeling their pelvis loosen and open up with this massage. When

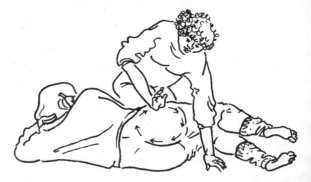

Lying on side for pelvic massage

one side feels well loosened up, ask her to roll over slowly on to the other side and loosen that up too. Concentrate on making the whole of the back of the hips feel free and open.

When you have finished give your friend time to rest and enjoy the sensation before she sits up again. Then change around. You don't have to be pregnant, or female, to enjoy the pleasures of massage!

CHAPTER 4

6-9 MONTHS

'I've had enough of this rent-a-body stuff,' said one 8½ months pregnant woman. You may well feel the same way as your pregnancy comes towards full term – and after 36 weeks you may get annoyed at the thought that your baby is surely just 'finishing off' the fancy bits like his fingernails and hair. In fact the last few weeks are important for your baby's health as he is laying down an extra fat layer which will keep him warm and help him fight infection, and he is also completing the development of his lungs so that he can breathe readily when born. So, even though you might well wish he would go away and do it somewhere else, your baby is doing some important final preparations for life outside the womb.

For you these 3 months are a time of hard work carrying your heavy baby, and also a time of approaching birth. As the date comes nearer it is not unusual to feel impatient and excited, but apprehensive as well. Whether you've had other babies or not, stage fright before birth is most understandable. The exercises in this chapter help you get ready to give birth. If it's too much sweat to clamber into a leotard or tracksuit let yourself off and do your exercises in a loose dress instead. Even if you feel fretful and uncomfortable have a go at them anyway. Oddly enough, stretching around can resettle your baby more comfortably in your pelvis and certainly alters your levels of seratonin and adrenalin for the better. Both these hormones affect your mood, and this is why exercise can so often cheer you up.

After the section of exercises for you alone is a set of massages for you to practise with your labour companion, and then some more breathing patterns to help you with your baby's birth. If you are joining the book at this stage of your pregnancy, read through the exercise sections in the other chapters first – some of the stretches have been decribed in detail earlier and so are described more briefly here. Although I've talked about the discomforts of the last weeks of pregnancy, there can also be pleasure luxuriating in the magnificence of your size and the generosity of your womb in making room for your child. Your movements, while slow, can be graceful and powerful.

STRETCH SESSION

Sit yourself down in a cleared space and cross your legs. Pull your bottom backwards a little to make sure you are sitting on the centre of your pelvic floor. Relax your hip, knee and ankle joints. Stretch your spine upwards and allow your shoulders to relax downwards. Allow your facial muscles to soften and relax, and steady your breathing down to a slightly slower rate than normal. Remind yourself that you are taking some time just for yourself, and use your breathing to calm yourself down. On the breath in, breathe in peace; on the breath out, breathe out tension. On the breath in, breathe in energy; on the breath out, breathe away tiredness. On the breath in, breathe in strength; on the breath out, breathe out fear. Let a quietness come.

Use any or all of these breathing exercises until you feel you have come to your centre. Remember throughout this session to make all efforts on a breath out, and to keep your face and throat relaxed. Then when you are ready, stretch your head, neck and shoulders as we have done before. With a well lifted spine and a steady rhythm of breathing:

1 Stretch your head forwards, chin on chest, head weighted by your linked hands. Come back up.

2 Stretch your head back, tipping your chin up. Stretch your throat by taking your lower lip over your upper lip a few times. Come back up.

3 Stretch your right ear to your right shoulder. Float your head back up.

4 Stretch your left ear to your left shoulder. Float your head back up.

5 Look over your right shoulder. Hold it. Look a little further. Come back to centre.

6 Look over your left shoulder. Hold it. Look a little further. Come back to centre.

7 Make slow circles with your head, twice to the right, then twice to the left.

8 Making sure your spine is still well lifted put your hands, palm to palm, behind your back; or hold opposite elbows, or opposite wrists, whatever is right for you.

9 Stretch one hand up between the shoulder blades, and catch it with the other (see p. 4). Then work the other way round.

10 Make a sitting twist (see p. 34) in both directions. Then stand up slowly. While you still feel like it, make standing stretches to the side (see p. 6) and to the front (see p. 17), then balance on each foot in turn in tree pose. If you feel like it you can go on doing these poses with great benefit right up until the birth. However, if you start to find these stretches too much, listen to your body, and leave them out for the time being.

On all fours practise these stretches to mobilize your hips and strengthen your wrists and arms (Figure 4.1). They are described in detail on p. 39. Move languorously and strongly in the rhythm of your breath.

1 Arch and flatten your back six times.

2 Make big circles with your hips, six to the right, six to the left.

3 Rock your hips backwards and forwards, taking your weight first more on your hands, then more on your knees.

4 Separate your knees and put your toes together. On a breath out stretch your bottom down towards your feet and your chest towards the floor. If you need some support put

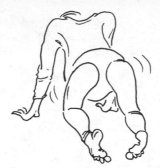

FIGURE 4.1

Transition rocking, all fours

a pile of pillows or cushions to go under your chest. Relax in this stretch for a minute or two.

Sitting on the floor, spread your legs as wide apart as you can. If you have been following the book all through your pregnancy you will notice a wider stretch by now. Put the backs of your hands on the fronts of your knees. Stretch the crown of your head towards the ceiling. On a breath out walk your hands forwards between your legs, stretching your chest downwards towards the floor. Don't worry if you can only stretch forward a few inches. Keep your back long. Don't squash your baby!

After three or four breaths in this position, breathe in and lift your head up, and breathing out, walk your hands back towards you and come back to centre.

Now put your feet sole to sole and bring them in towards your body (see p. 9). Bounce your knees very gently downward. Stretch them down to the floor if you can, but don't force them. Stay there while you take half-a-dozen slow, deep breaths. Feel your inner thighs loosen little by little. When you've finished gently lift your knees up with your hands and stretch your legs out in front of you.

Now practise squatting. Ease your heels towards the floor if you can, and if you can, press your knees further apart with your elbows – hands palm to palm. Both your inner thighs and your pelvic floor are well stretched in this position, and your pelvis is open to its widest. If you still need support to squat, hold on to the seat of a heavy chair, or alternatively perch your bottom on the edge of a few telephone directories or a fat dictionary. Do whatever's right for you.

Balance out all the opening of the thighs by turning them the other way in virasana (see p. 21). Kneel up and separate your feet. Sit down between your feet – if your knees are tight place a cushion between your feet. Linking your hands first with one index finger on the top, then the other, stretch your arms up above your head.

If you have become supple enough to lie back in virasana, you will find this very pleasant in the final weeks of pregnancy because it takes the pressure of the baby off your diaphragm. You will be doing pelvic squeezes every time you see the sticky stars on your walls (see p. 41) – but do half-a-dozen now just to make sure.

Now ease over on to your left side, one pillow under your head, another under your bent right knee. If you have practised 'savasana' (relaxation, or 'corpse pose') for many weeks, already your skill in 'letting go' will be precious to you by now (Figure 4.2). It's certainly not too late to learn it now though. Working from your feet up to your head, squeeze and release each group of muscles – feet, knees and calves, thighs, pelvic floor, buttocks, shoulders, hands and arms, mouth and face. On a breath in tighten a little; on a breath out let go profoundly. A sense of deep peace will come over you. Sink deeper and deeper into the floor. Let your imagination take you to a place you would like to be, whether a tropical beach, a peaceful garden, or your own personal landscape. While you relax feel your lower back spread and your pelvis open.

FIGURE 4.2

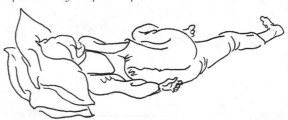

Relaxation on side

When you have had a little time to yourself place a hand on your tummy and say hello to your baby. From a tiny wisp of a thing she is now a great, strapping, robust individual. In the last few weeks a feeling of separateness begins to come between your personality and hers. This makes you look forward more to the birth and allows you not to be grieved at being parted by birth. Towards the end of pregnancy you can almost feel your baby say to you, 'Look here, I'm not you, I'm someone else, and it's about time I got out and really started to be that someone else.' Anyway, see what sort of communication seems to flow between the two of you.

When you've had enough you will feel your awareness slowly tuning in to your surroundings again. When you feel like it, ease yourself up by pressing your hands into the floor and sitting up.

CHOOSING A BIRTH

If you are using this book to be fit and strong, these exercises are enough. If you are preparing for an active birth, work your way through the next few pages too. If you aren't sure what kind of birth you'd like, have a look through the following section and see whether it helps you to decide. Any drugs you do use will interfere to some extent with your ability to move and breathe through your labour. Gas and air has the advantage over pethidine that if you have only used a little you can put the mask down and your system soon clears it. Pethidine is given in an injection and you can't get it out of your system if you change your mind! Give yourself the time and self-respect to work out what kind of birth is right for you. If you want a high-tech birth don't let earth-mother friends make you feel bad. If you want a passionate natural birth, stay with that even if your GP raises a quizzical eyebrow. Sort out whether any medical or policy difficulties will prevent you having your squatting delivery, or your epidural, or whatever, so that you know clearly where you stand.

TALKING TO STAFF

Any special wishes you have for the birth of your baby should be mentioned to your GP, to whoever you see at the ante-natal clinic and the midwife who comes to look after you as you arrive at the labour unit. Of these, the midwife who will be with you is the most important. Say quietly and firmly 'We're hoping to manage with a minimum of drugs', or 'We're hoping to manage without an episiotomy', or 'If all is well I'm hoping my baby can be delivered up on to my tummy.' Staff find 'we're hoping' less alienating than 'we shall' or 'we want'.

There are two main problems in the relationship between yourself and a midwife. One is that you will only have a baby a few times in your lifetime, and the midwife may deliver two or three every shift she works. She *can't* feel the intensity you do, although she's probably sincerely delighted by each baby's birth. The other is that you probably only meet when you are already in labour, and you have to have (or make) a rapport very quickly. If you really feel after an hour or so that the chemistry between you is impossible, get your companion to ask quietly and politely if you could be helped by someone else. Midwives themselves know only too well how important this rapport is. They will often quietly go away and arrange for someone else to replace them if they feel the relationship is not right. But if you do ask for a change of staff, do so quietly and with courtesy.

BREATHING FOR BIRTH

Sit cross-legged again to practise your breathing. If you feel very tired or floppy, support your back against a wall or the front of an armchair, or anything convenient.

Practise this abdominal breathing every day now. It will see you through almost all of your birth. You want it to be available to you automatically, any time you want it.

*1   Sit tall, spine lifting, shoulders relaxed. Place one
hand on your abdomen below your navel. Begin a slow and
steady rhythm of breathing.*
*2   When your slow rhythm has settled, start to breathe in
through your nose and out through your mouth. Keep
your mouth relaxed. Don't blow, just let the air escape
through your mouth.*
*3   When this is coming easily, send the breath in all the
way down to your hand. Let your tummy push your hand
out a little. Let the breath out come all the way up from
behind your hand. Let your tummy collapse back away
from your hand a little. The breath in is through the nose,
the breath out through the mouth. Continue this pattern
for a few minutes, then take your hand away from your
tummy, let your breathing return to its everyday level,
and blink your eyes open.*

BREATHING AND MOVING IN THE FIRST STAGE OF LABOUR

As the expected time for your baby's birth
approaches, practise these positions, combined with
the abdominal breathing described above, and a
rhythmic rocking and swaying of the hips. Your
practice of the exercises in this book will have made
you supple, strong and sensitive to the needs of
your unique body.

The first stage of labour may last anything from 3
to 16 hours or even longer. That is nothing like as
horrific as it sounds, since the really intense part will
probably be only from 4 to 8 hours. During this time
your cervix, the opening at the bottom of your
womb into your vagina, opens or 'dilates' from a
closed circle to a circle about 10 cm in diameter. Lay
a set of children's stacking beakers out in a row in
front of you. These are an enormous help in
visualizing what is going on inside. Your cervix is
closed when you start off, and through your first
stage dilates right up until it is as wide as the biggest
beaker! No wonder you feel something stupendous

is going on inside you. It is. Work out which beaker is about 4 cm across in diameter, which is 6 cm, which is 8 cm, etc. Then in your labour, if someone tells you you are 6 cm dilated, you can visualize how wide open you are. This is really encouraging.

Early contractions are like period pains, or you may feel them as twinges in your lower back, or buzzing cramp-like sensations in your thighs. The days before birth you will probably feel many of these tightenings as your uterus 'revs itself up' – and very confusing they are too; you really don't know if 'this is it' or not. Most labour wards ask you to call when you have had an hour of tightenings coming regularly every 5 minutes.

Handling the contractions of the last few days of pregnancy and the beginning of labour, you will suddenly appreciate the flexibility that has come from your yoga, and the awareness of yourself. You will also feel the benefit of your breathing skills. Let yourself feel good about the time and effort you've put in.

With these early contractions my strong recommendation is: don't do anything about them until you have to. See your labour as quite a long road stretching ahead of you and see how important it is not to use up all your mental and physical resources in the first few hours. So while you can handle your cramp-like contractions by relaxing your muscles, and perhaps by sliding easily into your slow, abdominal breathing, do so. Your body will tell you when you have to pay more attention to it.

When your contractions do ask for more of your attention try one of these positions:

1 Lean your head against the wall, knees bent. Combine abdominal breathing with swaying your hips in your own rhythm and relaxing and releasing everything from waist to knees (Figure 4.3). 'My god,' you will think to yourself, 'this works!' and it does. The sensation remains but much of the pain and tension goes away. Visualize your cervix opening up, fraction by fraction.

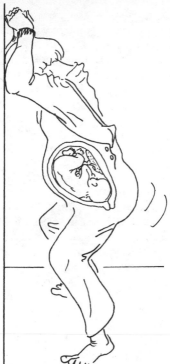

FIGURE 4.3

Arms, head on wall, hip sway

Or try this:
2   *Hold on to a windowsill, table top, or high hospital bed. Walk your feet back till your legs are vertical, your torso parallel to the floor. Relax your knees slightly and rock your hips, backwards and forwards, or round and round, and breathe slow and deep into your abdomen. In between contractions you will probably want to wander around doing bits and pieces if you're at home, or in hospital you may be encouraged to potter about and make cups of tea, or read, or chat. Your contractions will last less than a minute and be 3 or 4 minutes apart, so you definitely feel part of ordinary life in between them. These positions will probably do you very well until you are about 4 cm dilated.*

57

Things may begin to get more intense now. Contractions last longer, and are stronger. You need to concentrate on you. It's not rude not to answer a question in the middle of a contraction, nor to say quickly in between contractions 'I don't feel like chatting any more now'.

You may literally want to 'get down to it' more; your legs may not want to keep you standing up any longer. Try these positions for the middle part of the first stage as you go from about 4-7 cm dilated.

1   Kneel with your knees wide apart, your feet together. Rest on your hands or flop forwards on to a beanbag or a pile of pillows. When the contraction comes breathe steadily down into your abdomen. Move your hips in strong, slow movements, side to side, or backwards and forwards, or round in circles, whatever helps you. It's the movement in hips which is most important in staying with the contractions, and not fighting against them. In between contractions rest forwards *on to folded arms or a pile of pillows or a beanbag. Try to avoid being flat on your back.*
2   On all fours go with your contraction by breathing steadily into your abdomen. In this position you have great mobility in your hips. Rock and gyrate them strongly and smoothly. Be very relaxed in your pelvic floor.
3   Kneel up on a bed with your knees wide apart and your arms around a companion's neck. During contractions let yout thighs 'give' a bit and sway your hips. Breathe down into your abdomen. Keep your face soft and your jaw relaxed (Figure 4.4).

These suggestions are for guidance only. Use any, all or none of them when the time comes; invent your own variations; just listen to your body and do what it seems to need. Practise these positions, with the breathing and the hip-rocking, during the few weeks approaching birth, then they will all have become easy and familiar in case you want them.

The contractions grow from 0-7 cm of dilatation from a mild tightening cramp to a tremendous

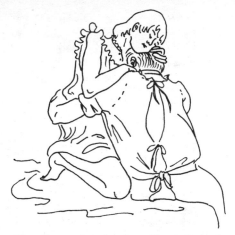

FIGURE 4.4

Kneeling up, arms round man's neck

surging 'rush' of sensation. For a few women there is no pain at all, but most of us experience some degree of pain and for many of us there's a great deal of it. Don't stop reading there! Preparation for childbirth has veered from my-poor-dear horror stories to 'conditioning' or 'training' methods which require one to 'detach' oneself from the pain using great willpower. I believe a better way, springing both from Sheila Kitzinger's psychosexual approach, and from Janet Balaskas, Mel Huxley and others of the Active Birth Movement, is to acknowledge that there may be pain, there may be great pain, but to be ready mentally and physically to use all possible physiological or 'natural' ways of dealing with it, and to go really positively into the experience. Many women do find they can ride the great waves of pain with strength: and then can enjoy the passion, the power and the triumph of their births.

Maybe this sounds way off your wavelength. If so, as I said at the beginning, you haven't been wasting your time with exercise: a fit body recovers better from a high-tech birth just as much as from a natural one.

Preparing to meet the stormiest part of most

labours, that is 7-10 cm dilation or the 'transition' phase, we will take a few minutes to work on one more 'natural' way of dealing with pain – using your voice. I am not talking about the wild cries of women stuck in hospital delivery rooms coping with births for which they weren't really prepared. I'm talking about using your voice to help yourself. Making a noise (like, incidentally, rhythmic swaying and deep abdominal breathing) raises in your body the levels of a substance called 'endorphin'. This is a natural secretion, something like morphine, which helps you cope with pain, but has the advantage of being something which, given the right circumstances, your body can produce for itself. If you feel yourself wanting to make a noise during 'transition' or 7-10 cm dilatation, try remembering these things:

1   Keep your mouth and throat relaxed.
2   Make the noise on a breath out.

Try this: squat and put one hand over your perineum. Now gasp in sharply, making a noise in your throat. Did you feel your pelvic floor pull up away from your hand? Now try this: groan in a deep voice on a slow breath out. Can you feel your pelvic floor open and bulge into your hand? Clearly its the second sort of noise we're going to choose since we're trying to open everything in the pelvis up.

Use this exercise to open up your voice.

VOICE EXERCISE

Sit cross-legged, spine lifting, shoulders relaxed. Close your eyes. Slow your breathing down and deepen it to the abdominal breathing we've practised. Now on your breaths out:

1   Make an 'mm' sound. Feel it vibrate in your lips and forehead. Do four or five of these.
2   Make an 'oo' sound. Feel it vibrate in your head and

throat. Do four or five.
3   Make an 'ah' sound. Feel your skull and ribcage
vibrate. Again do four or five.
4   Make a deep 'oh' sound. Feel your pelvis, ribcage and
skull all fill with the sound. Do four or five of these too.

You will probably notice, after the initial self-consciousness wears off, that your breaths get very deep and long and that you are making a marvellous noise. Groups of women trying this out will often get the giggles for a while then suddenly fall under its spell. Women who have given birth record that they used this 'chanting', 'crooning', 'singing-moaning' or even 'growling' to help them through the really tough parts of their labours.

BREATHING AND MOVING IN TRANSITION

Some women move through 7-10 cm dilatation quite smoothly and easily. For others of us it's quite a stormy time. Signs that transition are approaching are these: you may get the shivers, you may suddenly feel or be sick, you may suddenly change mood – from feeling brave and dynamic to angry and resentful, for instance. You may have one, or two, or all three of these signs. Your contractions will probably be enormous by now. They last 2½ minutes and are 3 minutes apart – say the books. Basically that means they are more or less continuous. You may well promise yourself or announce to the whole room that you will never, ever, ever, get yourself into this situation again. Try to remember somewhere in your mind that with any luck these last 3 cm are going to open up quite a lot quicker than the earlier 3 cm.

Keep your deep abdominal breathing going, using a deep resonant 'oh' or 'ah' on the outbreath if it helps. Try an all fours position where you can press your head hard into something. The comfort this gives is something like the comfort you get from

someone holding your head if you vomit (but in the
circumstances, a lot more profound). If you come on
to all fours you can push your head into your
companion's waist as he or she stands at the end of
the bed (Figure 4.5). They must be prepared to be
quite steady as you will burrow into them quite hard
at the height of your contraction. Sally wrote of this:

> I did not tell him at the time, but I felt as I pushed
> my head into him, Steve was a firm rock in the
> midst of an experience that threatened to over-
> whelm me.

Or Molly records:

> We knelt face to face and at the height of my
> contractions we pressed out foreheads together. I
> pressed my head against his really hard – then
> rested back on my heels in the short breaks.

FIGURE 4.5

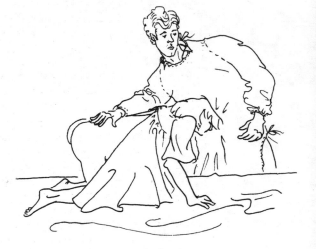

Head pushed into man's tummy

Through all this let your hips be free to move
during your contractions. Take any rests you get
between contractions in any position where you can
lean forwards with your thighs apart. Don't go flat
on your back. Rest on to pillows or a beanbag or a

friend. You may be angry at this time – or you may be scared. Acknowledge your anger or fear if you can. Say to it 'hello, I thought I'd meet you somewhere about now.' Don't let it drown you in a panic. Just stay with the process rather than fighting it and the anger and fear will pass.

Transition usually lasts somewhere between 10 minutes and an hour. It is coming to an end when you suddenly feel something different. What it feels most like is an urgent desire to empty your bowels. Indeed if there is anything in your bowels (if you didn't have diarrhoea or an enema or a suppository when you first arrived at the hospital), that is exactly what is going to happen next, so ask for a bedpan if you can get your breath. Whether you've got a full bowel or not, say to somebody 'I want to push'. If you and your companion are alone and 'getting on with it' get him or her to buzz the midwife now and tell her what is happening. She will do a vaginal examination. If your cervix is all dilated up to 10 cm she'll say 'you're fully dilated' or 'you can push now' and you know you are in the second stage.

If there is still a tiny rim of cervix left she will say 'don't push yet.' If you push on to an incompletely dilated cervix it may get puffy and swollen and that will make life much more difficult. So, allowing yourself a few choice curses, get into the knee-to-chest position. Your hospital gown, if you're wearing one, will part neatly over your bottom. Ignore it! When contractions come breathe steadily down into your abdomen and rock your hips. Both these things will help your cervix to stretch up the last little bit. When you feel like pushing, change your breathing to a fast 'huff huff BLOW, huff huff BLOW; huff huff BLOW', and as the urge goes away change back to slow breathing. Relax between contractions as much as you can. Knee-to-chest is the best way to slow down any labour that is going too fast because you tip the weight of the baby off the cervix. If, for instance, you're still at home and feel things are progressing frighteningly fast, alert the hospital, ring your partner or friend or the ambulance to tell them you need your lift, *unlock the door*, then get into the knee-to-chest position and try to calm yourself down.

Eventually, either your midwife will say 'Great - you're fully dilated now,' or you will suddenly KNOW that there is *nothing in the world* that can stop you pushing. (This means you're fully dilated.) When you have a rim of cervix left you can resist the urge to push – only just, but you can resist it. When you are fully dilated, if someone came in and said you would be beheaded at dawn if you pushed, you would *still* push! Sooner or later, one way or another your cervix will be 10 cm dilated, as wide open as the biggest beaker in the stacking set, and your baby's head will be ready to move into your vagina. After negotiating the stormy seas of transition you will suddenly come back into the world again. You are ready to push your baby out into the world. Or as one woman said after a heavy transition, 'Baby? Oh yes – I'd forgotten there was going to be a *baby*!'

FIGURE 4.6

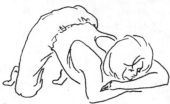

Knee-to-chest – can slow things down

POSITIONS AND BREATHING FOR SECOND STAGE

Sometimes, if there is an emergency, it's necessary to have your feet in stirrups and to push your baby out lying on your back, to allow the staff maximum view and ease of manoeuvre. But, if there is no emergency, this is about the worst position to get into for your baby to be born. Depending on the policy of your hospital or nursing home, it may be a good idea to talk about this with your midwife or doctor first. (See the section on 'Talking with staff', p. 54.) The chances are that you will know instinctively what feels right to you at the time. Squatting, all fours, kneeling upright so your baby is born 'forwards', or kneeling and inclining your upper body forwards so your baby is born 'back-wards' (almost like all fours) are all useful.

In the second stage there are often longer pauses between the contractions, which start with the usual 'contraction' feeling, and then develop into a huge and powerful desire (and desire is the word) to bear down. Here is the best way to practise pushing:

PRACTISING PUSHING

(empty your bladder before you do this)
Squat down and put one hand on the floor to help you balance. Put the other hand on your pelvic floor. Breathe steadily into your abdomen. Now imagine a desire to push, and your baby's head, the size of a good-sized grapefruit sitting up in the top of your vagina. Take a deep breath in. As you breathe out release your pelvic floor, really bulge your perineum into your hand – and imagine pushing the grapefruit-sized head downwards strongly and powerfully, until the breath is finished. Keep your mouth relaxed, also your jaw and your throat. Another breath in, and repeat the strong deep push, down in your pelvis. Keep your perineum bulging into your hand. Push as long as the breath lasts. Another breath in, and on the breath out another long, powerful push. Then relax. Most of your contractions will have a pushing urge long enough for you to take two or three breaths and make two or three good pushes. When you practise imagine the head moving downwards a little as you push, and easing back a fraction as you breathe in. This slow squeezing downwards, with a little easing back after each push, gives the tissues of your vagina time to stretch open. You may not want to push very strongly while you practise – that's fine – just get the

hang of co-ordinating the breath, letting go of the pelvic floor, and then imagine using the power of the contraction to push the baby's head downwards. If you don't empty your bladder before you start you're likely to wet yourself – but at least you know you're doing it right if that happens!

FIGURE 4.7

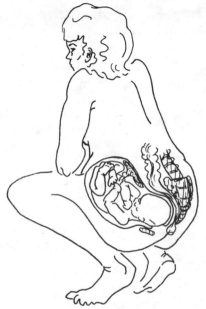

Head of baby presses rectum, etc.

A couple more useful thoughts about this: (as your baby's head slides down your vagina there will probably be a few contractions where you feel a really shocking, preposterous pressure on your *back* passage (Figure 4.7). You can see from the figure that the baby is pressing right on to it, and that is why you feel this. Keep your pelvic floor relaxed. In a few more minutes the head will get 'round the bend' and be sitting behind the opening of the vagina waiting to be born at last.

Use all of your body's surge of power while you push, and use a deep 'oh' or 'ah' on the outbreath again if it helps. You won't get a sore throat if you sing or chant the sound with your throat relaxed.

You can reach your cervix with the tip of your middle finger. So you only have to push your baby, all in all, about the length of that middle finger.

PRACTISING FOR THE CROWNING OF THE HEAD

The thoughts of something the size of a baby in your vagina may be disheartening if you have spent years struggling to push tampons in uncomfortably. However, your vagina is not always as tight and dry as it is when you're trying to get a tampon in, perhaps in a hurry. If it doesn't embarrass you, try sliding a finger inside your vagina sometime when you're very turned on, and notice how soft and stretchy and slippery it becomes. The conditions inside your vagina are quite similar to this when you are in labour. Can you feel all the complicated folds of tissue inside your vagina? All those can unfold, spread out, and stretch, to make room for your child.

When the baby's head is at last at the entrance to the vagina the midwife will ask you to 'pant, not push' so that the head is born slowly, giving your delicate tissues enough time to spread out and allow the head through without injury. What will this part of the birth feel like? Women describe a burning or stretching sensation in their vagina – and a feeling of complete disbelief. 'This is quite impossible!'

Put several fingers in your mouth and stretch your lips very wide. Notice the uncomfortable, hot, stretching feeling. Now take your fingers out and notice that your mouth is not hurt in any way. That is very like the feeling you will feel in your vagina as the head 'crowns' or eases through. Practise it several times in the last weeks of pregnancy so you are well used to it and, when you feel it down in your vagina, can recognize what is going on.

67

Practise the crowning by squatting and putting one hand on the floor to help you balance. Put the other hand over your perineum. Bulge your perineum down warmly into your hand. Now imagine your baby's grapefruit-sized head is resting just behind the entrance to your vagina. Imagine your midwife saying 'with your next contraction, pant, don't push'. Release your pelvic floor even more, and pant – butterfly-light panting – jaw relaxed, eyes soft. Imagine that ridiculous, enormous, hot stretch of your vagina. Keep open, keep panting. It will take at least 4 or 5 seconds for the head to slide out. Now relax, and rest. Try this out often as the time for the birth comes near. It will be a terrific help when your baby is born.

When you're giving birth, you may feel at maximum stretch that you want to shout. Women the world over do this. If you want to, keep your pelvic floor relaxed, throw your head back, and give a shout! There is a connection between the vagina and the throat, and it may be that a single yell opens your throat and lets your vagina open a fraction more. Don't feel you *ought* to do this – but if it comes instinctively, be aware that a great many women do it. Your instinct may be to be serene, or determined, or dignified, or very animal: whatever your instinct is will be what is right for you.

Sometimes books make it sound as though once the head's been born the birth is more or less over. Don't stop concentrating because the shoulders are quite big and you need to stay relaxed to ease them out. Many midwives are really helpful with this and will guide you by saying 'give a gentle push – now pant – now another little push – pant again' and so on, while first one shoulder, then the other is born. Throughout all this keep your mouth and eyes relaxed, and keep your pelvic floor releasing downwards. Work through this part of the birth in your imagination too.

After the shoulders are born the rest of the baby slithers out and will be lying there, wriggling away, with little thrashing limbs. Until he breathes he will be quite blue in colour. Once he starts to breathe he will turn to a lovely pink colour. He may have patches of creamy 'vernix' on his skin – the substance which stopped his skin getting dried out by the water he has lived in all these months.

If your baby needs any help breathing his mouth or nose will be suctioned with tiny tubes or he might be given a little oxygen. He will be wiped and weighed then wrapped up and given to you.

If you would like your baby to be delivered straight up on to your tummy if all is well with him and you, tell the staff about this and in most hospitals now they will be very happy to do this.

MASSAGE AND HELP IN LABOUR

Try out these massages with your labour companion. For early first stage:

Stand and put your arms round your companion's neck as though you were dancing with her, or him (Figure 4.8). Your partner should reach round to your lower back and massage it with strong slow circles, while you practise a 'contraction' – letting your knees 'give' a little, rock or sway your hips, and breathe deeply into your abdomen.

For the middle of first stage:

You kneel up on a bed and put your arms round your companion's neck. Again let him or her reach round to your lower back and massage it firmly while you breathe and rock your way through a contraction (see Figure 4.4).

Also have your companion massage your back while you kneel with your knees apart and feet together and you lean forwards. Have a 'contraction' and rock and breathe so that your companion has a chance to get used to how you will sound and look.

Let the companion sit with his or her legs apart, knees bent. You sit snuggled up to him or her. Push the back of your hips into him or her. As your

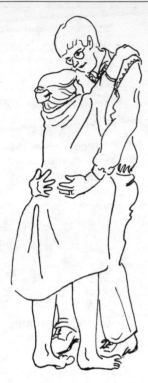

FIGURE 4.8

Standing backrub

contraction starts let your companion rock you from side to side with his or her knees while you do your abdominal breathing (Figure 4.9). This feels very comforting.

For transition

Look at Figures 4.4 and 4.5. Try out these positions and in both of them imagine a really strong 2 or 2½ minute contraction and push your head really quite hard.

Just as important, talk together about what it might be like to go through this intense and difficult part of the labour together. Share your thoughts and worries and make sure you understand each other's desires and needs as you plan to get through this part of your baby's birth.

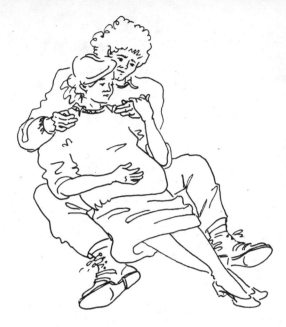

FIGURE 4.9

Sitting 'spoons'

For second stage

Your companion can support you on one side as you squat on a bed, or can support you from behind as you squat on the floor. Find out before you go into labour whether your hospital will accept you doing this, if the 'supported squat' (made famous by films and photographs of Michel Odent's clinic in Pithiviers) is a position you feel you would like (Figure 4.10).

Otherwise your companion can help you by simply being near and holding, touching, or just talking to you in any way you would like him or her to.

Helping with breathing

Get your companion to do some abdominal breathing with you so that he or she knows what it's like. It's very useful in any stressful situation and is a skill everyone can use – so it's useful for him or her to learn it for their own benefit as well as yours.

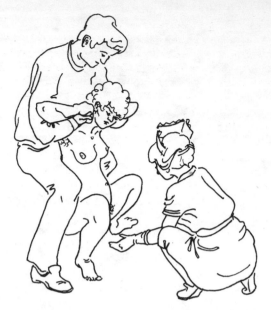

Supported squat

Explain to your companion that this breathing may become noisy but that you are using it to focus within, and to go with the opening-up process of your contractions rather than fighting them. Your friend or partner's most useful role is to remind you to breathe *out*. When you are concentrating hard, or trying hard, or under pressure, you may notice that you breathe in hard, but forget to breathe out fully, so get into a cycle of shallow breathing and gasping. Remembering always to give a good, slow, deep breath out will ensure that you stay in a cycle of slow, deep breaths. Ask them to be ready to say quietly to you 'breathe out' if you hold your breath, and if you don't hear or understand them because you are concentrating so hard, to blow quietly near your ear (not into it!) – this will lead you instinctively to breathe out yourself.

Show your friend or partner the knee-to-chest position and the huff-huff-BLOW breathing which you will use if you want to push before your cervix is fully open. Then if you forget it in the heat of the moment your partner can remind you. Explain to your partner that if you want to change position in strong labour you may need physical help. It can feel very difficult to get from, say, all fours into a squat when you are in powerful labour.

NOTES TO LABOUR COMPANIONS

Do remember that labour often takes many hours. Pace yourself – don't use up all your compassion and energy in the first couple of hours. Look after your own body. Be careful how you stretch your back if you are doing a lot of back massage or taking a lot of the woman's weight (for instance, if she has her arms around your neck, as in Figure 4.3). Stuff a couple of chocolate bars into your pocket on the way out (if you've got time to organise it take some sandwiches and a thermos of tea or coffee) in case you suddenly feel hungry yourself.

Take time to talk over with the person who is giving birth:

1 How will we feel when labour starts? How will you get in touch with me? How will we decide when to go into hospital?
2 How will we work together through the early first stage? Through the middle part of the first stage? How will we handle transition? What will it be like for us?
3 How will pushing be? How can I best help you here?
4 What do you feel about using drugs? (For an excellent brief description of the effects of the drugs usually offered, see Angela Phillips with Nicky Lean and Barbara Jacobs, *Your Body, Your Baby, Your Life*, pp. 128–34.) Make sure you understand exactly what the woman giving birth feels about this and what signal or word she can give you if she really changes her mind during labour.

By talking these things through you will work out at least what the emotions you anticipate will be.

Here, though, is the most important note of all. As a labour companion you must be as flexible as you possibly can. No birth is like any other birth. Even if you have been with this same person during other births, this experience may be quite different from the others. Some women who love to cuddle and stroke generally don't want to be touched *at all* during labour. This is not a rejection of you – it is simply how that particular labour goes. Other women need constant massage and can hardly bear to let their companion go for 30 seconds to have a pee! You can't tell in advance what it's going to be like. The range of emotions you go through together may move from excitement to despair to elation. Labour may be serene, or it may be dramatic. You've simply got to be ready to be as sensitive and instinctive as you can in your responses, preparing yourself by really letting yourself know beforehand what a powerful process labouring and giving birth can be. Although she will probably be too occupied to tell you until afterwards, the caring presence of someone like you is the most fantastic help (and the most powerful anaesthetic!) that a birthing woman can have.

CHAPTER 5

BIRTH DAYS

STARTING OFF

JENNIE: 'I noticed my 'Braxton Hicks' contractions were becoming rather regular – and by the time we were shopping in Mothercare I was longing to get down on my hands and knees and sway my hips.'

SARA: 'My waters broke in bed just as my husband said they would. He had little time to gloat. . . .'

JENNIFER (2am): 'I stood at the top of the stairs saying 'Oh my goodness, this is more than every 5 minutes', and my husband stood at the bottom of the stairs, saying 'Get dressed, get dressed'.

GETTING THERE

CATHY: 'I knelt on the floor in the back of the taxi and rested my head and arms on the seat.'

JENNIFER: 'We tipped the front passenger seat forwards and I travelled in the back of the car. I couldn't get comfortable and crawled up and down.'

FIRST STAGE

SUZANNE: 'Swaying my hips was marvellous – any sensation of pain and tension disappeared as I rocked.'

SARA: 'I leaned on the windowsill and looked outside. It meant a lot to see people doing ordinary things like gardening. . . .'

CHRIS: 'I sprawled on to the marvellous beanbags.'

Sometimes there's a lot of backache

FIGURE 5.1

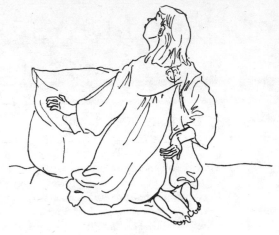

'Oh my *pigging* back!'

Sometimes first stage takes ages and ages

FIGURE 5.2

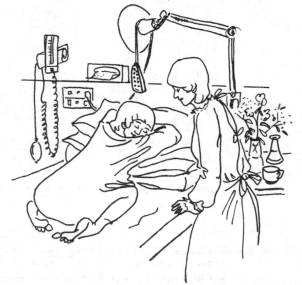

'Wake me up if anything happens'

FIGURE 5.3

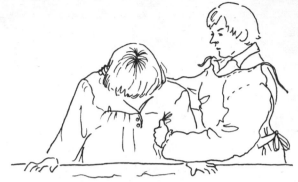

'Is it Wednesday or Thursday?'

and attendants become weary too

FIGURE 5.4

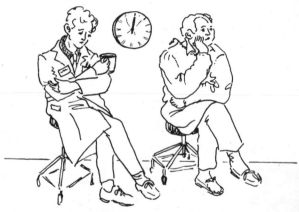

'This is going to be a Friday's child' (husband and medical student)

Some first stages are fast, or happen almost without you knowing

ROSE: 'I woke up with strong contractions and thought 'Oh Lord, if this is what it's like at the beginning, I don't think I'm going to do it very well at all' – but when I got to hospital I was already 9 cm dilated!'

LOUISE: 'It must have been while I was in the bath that I

77

moved into second stage, but I didn't realize this at the time. We arrived at hospital and told sister I was pushing!'

Transition can be a suprise

SARA: 'My legs became shaky and I giggled to myself as I thought I couldn't be in transition yet!' (she was)

or overwhelmingly powerful

HELEN: 'I couldn't believe I could contain so much sensation. It was like going down the middle of a whirlpool.'

 FIGURE 5.5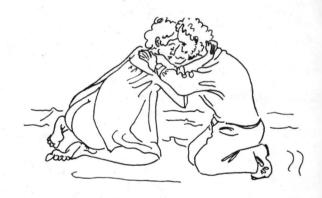

'Hold on to me'

ANN (URGENTLY): 'Hold me then.'

and waiting to push is very hard

HELEN: 'oh damn, damn, damn, damn, DAMN!'

At last it's time to push

FIGURE 5.6

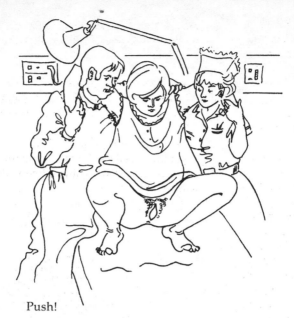

Push!

HUSBAND: 'Isn't she *strong*.'

FIGURE 5.7

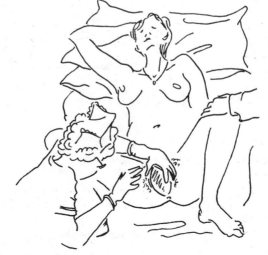

Pant. The head crowns

FIGURE 5.8

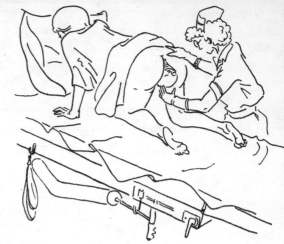

Head born, all fours

'Pant, don't push'

FIGURE 5.9

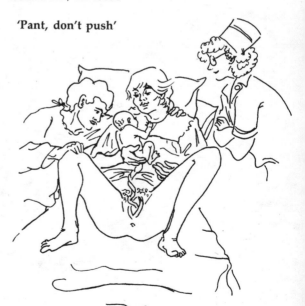

Suddenly..! Baby, cord, on tummy

and at last here's your baby.

FIGURE 5.10

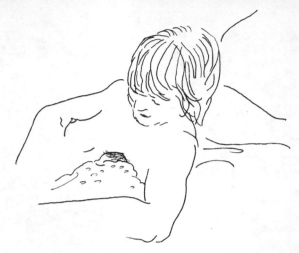

Christina holds Emily to breast

CAROLE: 'words cannot describe how you feel when you finally see your baby after all those months growing inside you.'

FIGURE 5.11

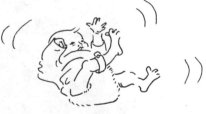

Baby – dressed!

CHAPTER 6

IF THINGS GO WRONG

It is sad to have this chapter here, but we must respect that for some women pregnancy does not end happily. Rarely nowadays, but still for a few people, birth ends with a baby's death, or with the birth of a handicapped child. Also, there is sometimes something wrong with a pregnancy such that the baby is lost long before the end of the 9 months. Please don't read this chapter at all if your pregnancy is going well and you feel it will upset you. It is here because women going through such losses are sad and angry to find themselves 'shut out' suddenly from all their books about babies and birth – and also to remind those of us close to anyone going through such a loss, that our support and our ability to listen generously are what they need most of all.

A brief guide to information, helplines, and a few suggestions to aid your recovery are included in this chapter. For a detailed and compassionate book including lots of accounts written by women themselves about their experiences of miscarriage, see *Miscarriage* by Ann Oakley *et al*. Fontana, 1984. For support and advice about the experience of loss, see the chapters on 'Loss and Grieving' in Sheila Kitzinger's *Women's Experience of Sex*, and her chapters about the loss of babies in *Pregnancy and Childbirth*. Look too at Susan Borg and Judith Lasker's book, *When Pregnancy Fails*, Routledge & Kegan Paul, 1982, for other women sharing their feelings about miscarriage.

WHAT CAN GO WRONG

Ectopic pregnancy

In an ectopic pregnancy, the fertilized egg does not manage to get all the way down the fallopian tube before it starts trying to implant itself. The pregnancy therefore begins to develop in one of the two tubes leading into your womb instead of in your womb itself, and there is not room for it, nor can enough nourishment get to it. Signs of an ectopic pregnancy are a bad pain on one side low down in the abdomen, and sometimes vaginal bleeding too. If you get a bad pain low down in your abdomen on one side, and it is 2 or 3 weeks after a missed period and you could be pregnant, get in touch with your doctor.

If it is early in the pregnancy, sometimes the foetus can be removed and the tube repaired afterwards. Otherwise the tube itself may have to be removed.

After an ectopic pregnancy, discuss with your doctor why it happened and whether your chances of conceiving again are affected.

Miscarriage

A baby for whom you have waited, of whom you were very aware almost as soon as she was conceived, is a very real person to you. Should you lose that person even after a very few weeks you need to allow yourself space and time to grieve over her.

A miscarriage before 12 weeks of pregnancy feels at first like the beginning of a period. Low in your abdomen you may have period-like cramps, and you will start to lose blood. Any vaginal bleeding in pregnancy could be the start of a miscarriage – contact your doctor at once. She will probably tell you to go to bed and rest and it is possible that the bleeding will stop and the pregnancy will continue safely. If, however, the miscarriage is 'inevitable', that is, if the baby has died or has not developed properly in some way, the loss will continue. Contact the doctor again if the bleeding does not stop within a few hours and find out what to do next.

A miscarriage later in pregnancy may involve many hours of contractions. It is terribly hard to come to terms with the loss of a small person who has been kicking around inside you. Be as gentle with yourself as you can; give yourself time to think, talk and cry yourself through your feelings.

Staff at the hospital will be careful to make sure you see the baby if you want to, or to protect you from seeing the baby if you feel it would be too distressing. It really is up to you. Even if you don't want to see the baby it might be useful to know the sex – it can be easier to grieve over someone whose sex you know. But again, that is not a rule. If you think it will only increase your pain to know more, don't feel you have to ask.

If you think it would help you to get in touch with other women who have also experienced miscarriage write to The Miscarriage Association, Dolphin Cottage, 4 Ashfield Terrace, Thorpe, Nr, Wakefield, West Yorks, WF11 9QH.

Losing a baby around the time of birth

Sadly, some babies die shortly before, or shortly after, birth. About one in 3,000 babies every year are lost this way in the UK. It is for the parents what one midwife describes as 'a massive, horrible experience', and you will need time, support and love to find a way of living with it.

You will want to know, if possible, why your baby has died. Make an appointment to see your consultant and discuss the results of any post mortem examination, to find out whether there was a clear medical reason.

It might help to talk to other parents who have lost babies just before or just after birth. You can contact them through the Stillbirth and Neonatal Death Association, 37 Christchurch Hill, London NW3 1LA.

Medical abortion

If your pregnancy has to be ended for medical

reasons this may well be in the middle of the pregnancy when you are already very involved with your child and have felt him moving inside you. It is a hard experience to go through. Afterwards you will need to grieve the loss of this child just as much as if it had been a late miscarriage.

A handicapped child

You may know from ante-natal diagnosis that you will have a handicapped baby, or you may not know till the birth, or even some months later. The shock and complicated feelings you may well experience need to be respected. Use the resources of your consultant, GP, midwife and health visitor to find out as much as you can, and contact the support group which can give you most support and advice.

Association for Spina Bifida and Hydrocephalus,
Tavistock House North,
Tavistock Square,
London WC1H 9HJ.
01-380 0291

Down's Children Association,
4 Oxford Street,
London W1N 9FL.
01-580 0511

MENCAP (Royal Society for Mentally Handicapped Adults and Children),
123 Golden Lane,
London EC1Y ORT.
01-253 9433

Spastics Society,
12 Park Crescent,
London W1N 4EQ.
01-636 5020

Guilt

It's very common to feel guilty after a miscarriage, a stillbirth or neonatal death, or after the birth of a handicapped child. It's extremely rare for anything you did to cause any of these tragedies. Neither sexual intercourse, nor argument, cause miscarriage, although if a miscarriage happens after either of those things it may feel to you as though they did. It's very unlikely that anything you did caused your baby's handicap.

Try to find somebody (health visitors are often marvellous) with whom you can talk about feelings of guilt so that you don't get swamped.

Letting go

One day all of us will die. Everybody we love has to die one day. In our present culture we are ill-accustomed and ill-prepared for taking in and thinking about these facts. This makes it even harder to cope with a miscarriage or a stillbirth when somebody we loved, perhaps even from 5 or 6 weeks of pregnancy, and hardly had time to name or know, dies.

The love for all our children must include an ability, when it becomes necessary, to let the child go. With a living and healthy child we have 15 to 20 years gradually to let her go before she leaves home. With the loss of a baby we have to do it in hours or even minutes. However, it is still an aspect of our love for the child to be able to let her go when we have to, and it is that act of 'letting go' which allows parents who have lived through such a tragedy to move, finally, through the darkness and back into the light.

FIGURE 6.1

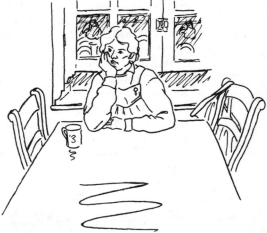

It is terribly hard to come to terms with the loss of a small person . . .

CHAPTER 7

THE FIRST 2 WEEKS AFTER BIRTH

Don't panic! Or rather, don't panic about panicking. In the first couple of weeks after your baby's birth you may feel as though you experience just about every emotion there is. Joy and excitement is sometimes followed after 36 or 48 hours by a flood of tears. Sometimes the tears are to do with sore stitches, sore breasts when your milk comes in, homesickness if you're in hospital, exhaustion if you're at home. Some people think you just have to have a big cry because your hormones are readjusting after the birth, and some people feel it's because the climax of birth is bound to be followed by an anti-climax and the realization of total responsibility for this helpless new being, plus the feeling that life will never be 'free' and the same again. Whatever the reason it's confusing and upsetting for you to be weeping when you think you 'ought' to be happy. But let the tears come; there are only a finite amount of them and after another day or two they will simply pass. Explain to perplexed partners and friends that you just feel vulnerable and over-whelmed if you don't want to dig around for reasons. Not everybody has the blues like this, but quite a lot of women do.

A much more serious kind of depression hits some women after the birth of their babies. It tends not to start until a little longer after the birth, and is not characterized by a day or two of weeping, but by a long time (sometimes months) of crying, anxiety, a dreadful blank feeling inside. Of course we all feel those things intermittently, but for some suffering from post-natal depression it just seems to go on and on, day in, day out. If you feel this way, tell someone, get help. Don't be ashamed and feel no one will understand. Tell your health visitor, your GP, your partner, and get assistance. If you can't talk to those people, or indeed if ever you feel you can't go on, if you can get to a phone, ring the Samaritans. You don't have to be on the verge of suicide to ring them, and they offer real listening and a chance to sort your feelings out a bit before you decide to talk to anybody else. Find out if there is a local post-natal support group.

YOUR BODY AFTER BIRTH

After your baby is born you will lose blood from your vagina for 2 or 3 weeks. For the first few days this flow of blood is really quite heavy – like the height of a heavy period or even more. You'll wear sanitary towels to deal with this as tampons would introduce a risk of infection. If you had a tear or an episiotomy you may feel tender around the stitches, and if you had a forceps birth you may be generally quite bruised inside.

As soon as it crosses your mind and you feel you can after your baby is born, give your pelvic floor a gentle squeeze or two.

Your breasts 'fill up' with milk 3 or 4 days after your baby is born. At first the baby gets colostrum from your breasts – this clear liquid doesn't look impressive but contains substances that will help your baby resist infection and disease. The baby only needs a very little of this in the first few days. After 3 or 4 days you find fountains of milk pouring from your breasts. It takes a while for your body to work out how much to produce and it tends to overdo it at first! For a few days your breasts may be hot, tight and full to the limit. 'Like rocks' and 'like concrete' is how many women women describe their breasts at this time. Ice cubes wrapped in clean tea towels or nappies and applied to the worst aches can help, as, if you're desperate, can getting into a hot bath and letting your breasts float in the water and letting the milk stream out. Expressing milk only encourages your breasts to make more, so don't do that unless you really can't stand it any longer.

After another 3 or 4 days your breasts will probably settle down, and make only the amount of milk your baby needs. If you go on producing an abundance then ring the hospital and see if they have a 'milk bank' or your local NCT who often supervise such a scheme. Breast milk is the very best food for premature babies and they may like to come and collect spare milk from you if you have it. A midwife or NCT person would call and explain to you how to collect and refrigerate your excess milk if you were going to join such a scheme.

Looking at your tummy may be the hardest part of all. A few lucky or tremendously fit women deflate instantly after their babies are born, and 2 or 3 days later zip themselves casually into their pre-baby jeans. Most of us gaze in amazement at the wobbly pouch that remains. Try to remember if you are sitting in the bath a few days after your baby's birth looking down at huge engorged breasts and a squashy tummy, and crying bitterly over your estranged body, that you really are not alone. Most of us do exactly that. Also try to remind yourself of your body's capacity for transformation and strengthening itself. As the milk calms down the breasts subside, and as you first rest and recover, then begin doing post-natal exercises. The muscle tone in your abdomen will come back and the abdomen can become flat and tight again.

Try to travel through this leaky, achey few days or weeks being gentle with yourself. Don't hate your body. It is doing a marvellous job of recovery and renewal. Rest it, love it, give it a chance, and you will be able to widen your experience and understanding of your physical self in many ways. Soon you will feel like the old familiar you again, with a lot of new knowledge and insight as well.

A practical point – take loose clothes to hospital for your 'going home' clothes and clothes that you can breastfeed in. It is horrible getting hot and bothered trying to squeeze yourself into some outfit that really doesn't fit yet.

EXERCISES FOR 0-14 DAYS

'Savasana' or 'corpse pose', the deep relaxation you've now practised for many months (see p. 10), and the most important exercise you can do during this 2 weeks. Collect everything you need for you and your baby into one room so that you aren't running around the house all day, and settle yourself down. Don't worry about 'getting back to normal'; treat yourself as a birthing kind of person for a good 2 weeks, and do 10 or fifteen minutes of complete relaxation every chance you get. Sometimes do your relaxation lying on your tummy (a long-awaited pleasure!) so that the gentle pressure this puts on your abdomen helps your womb to contract back down to its non-pregnant size, which it miraculously does within 6 weeks.

Never worry that while you are relaxing you are 'doing nothing'. You are doing the very best work towards regenerating your energy, and your identity, and getting ready for your new life.

Fit in these other exercises a few times every day if you can.

HIP ROCKING

Lying on your back in bed, draw your knees up. Inhale deeply. As you exhale pull your tummy button towards your spine; push your lower back into the bed and rock your hips up towards you. Inhaling, relax, then exhaling, rock your hips up again. Notice how the abdominal and buttock muscles tighten as you rock, and let go as you relax down. Rock your hips half-a-dozen times in the rhythm of your own steady breathing. Do two or three lots of half-a-dozen rocking exercises every day. You will notice how your muscles respond only a tiny bit on the first day after birth, but by the fifth or sixth day make a far stronger action.

BUTTOCK MUSCLES

Lie on your back in bed. Inhale deeply. As you exhale squeeze your buttock muscles strongly. Inhaling, relax them again. With this exercise too, do two or three sets of half-a-dozen exercises each day.

PELVIC FLOOR

Lying in bed, bend your legs up and separate your feet and knees a little. Inhale, and as you breathe out squeeze the muscles of your pelvic floor. Hold for a little while if you can, breathing steadily, then on another breath out relax. Do two or three sets of six pelvic floor squeezes every day.

Sometimes for a day or two after birth nothing happens when you try to tighten your pelvic floor! Don't panic – just try the exercise out a couple of times each day, and usually by the sixth or seventh day you'll get a response.

If you have stitches in your vagina, squeezing these muscles aids the healing process by improving blood circulation in the area. However, don't force yourself if you feel too tender. Waiting a few days before you start to exercise these muscles won't do any harm.

FEET AND ANKLES

To keep the circulation moving in your legs while you are resting for long periods of time, point and flex each foot half-a-dozen times, and circle each foot from the ankle half-a-dozen times, two or three times a day.

HEAD, NECK AND SHOULDERS

Do the familiar sequence of head, neck and shoulder stretches (described on p. 2) at least once every day. The new positions you need to get into to breastfeed may make you stiff and sore in these areas if you don't keep easing them out.

While your baby is tiny try one or even two pillows on your lap for your baby to rest on while you feed, so that you can relax your shoulders. Or try putting pillows by your side, on the side you are going to feed, and cuddle your baby to you under your arm, in order to ease stiffness from repeatedly getting into the more usual feeding posture (Figure 7.1).

FIGURE 7.1

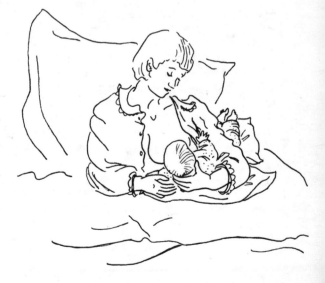

Feeding baby under arm

When you are tired support your back well so that your spine doesn't slump while you're feeding your baby. Collapsing your back will tend to give you aches and pains all over your body, so it really is worth remembering, in the midst of everything else, to keep your spine as long and supple as you can.

CO-COUNSELLING

In the early days with a new baby it is important to allow your feelings to evolve, rather than feeling under pressure to make statements of intent.

'It won't make any difference to my life.' 'Of course I'm going back to work.' 'Of course I'm not going back to work.' 'I'm so happy being a mother.' 'I'm so miserable being a mother,' are all sweeping statements made by women who feel under pressure to define themselves, their lives, their futures, within days of giving birth to their babies. 'Isn't it all gorgeous. Aren't you lucky?' says one lot of friends. 'You're comletely tied down now! How can you stand it?' says another lot. Pulled in both directions, intruded on by both views, you don't know how you feel, where you stand.

If possible set aside some time once or twice a week with a trusted and reliable friend who won't press *her* views, or with your partner, to talk about your new feelings and experiences in an exploratory way. Find out what you need and want to do with your time and responsibilities. Talk about what you're enjoying and what you're hating. Talk about how life with your baby matches or doesn't match with your hopes and expectations beforehand.

When you've had time to yourself to explore your feelings, you can in return give to your co-counselling partner some time to explore some issue which is important in their lives at the moment.

CHAPTER 8

2 WEEKS-
3 MONTHS AFTER
THE BIRTH

For several weeks after your baby's birth, days where you have abundant energy may alternate with waves of exhaustion. These swings up and down in energy gradually level out, and by the time your baby is 7 or 8 months old you will probably feel as though your energy cycle is back to normal again. It may be sooner than 7 months, or later than 8, depending on how often the baby wakes at night. If you ever find yourself crying with tiredness, although this isn't unusual, it is a signal you must listen to. Try to sleep during the day while your baby sleeps for the next 2 or 3 days. Should you find yourself in tears with tiredness all the time you must get some help – share some chores with someone else if you can. If there's no-one to share with, contact your health visitor and tell her you are in need of some support. Tell all visitors, friends and family that they can only visit if they bring with them food – fresh or pre-cooked ready to put in the oven.

Have a go at doing your exercises on tired days as well as energetic ones, because a good stretch out and a bit of time to yourself can make you less rather than more tired. Do your stretches while your baby sleeps after a feed or while someone else is available to listen out for her while you have a bit of time to concentrate on you.

You may be impatient now to really repossess your body – to lose the soft curves of pregnancy and the days immediately following birth, to feel your hips, thighs and upper arms back to their normal size again, and your tummy muscles resilient and strong.

As far as diet goes, stay off cakes, sweets and sweet fizzy drinks, but do not go short of essential foods. You need them to complete your recovery and to fuel you for your busy new life. Try to make sure you have fresh fruits and vegetables for vitamins and minerals, and protein in the form of pulses (lentils, etc.), cheese, eggs, meat or fish. Fill up with baked potatoes or wholemeal bread.

If you managed to give up smoking don't start again! Think of all the places you might be able to afford to take your baby to, from the swimming pool, perhaps even on holiday, if you don't start throwing your money to the tobacco companies again. Think of all the games and running around with your child you'll be able to enjoy so much more if you're not coughing and spluttering. If you've used cigarettes as rewards in the past, try to think of other ways of being nice to yourself. If you could choose to do the best thing for your baby's body – not smoking – can you choose to do the best thing for yours? Furthermore, babies growing up with smokers are much more prone to coughs, colds and illness.

As for exercise, try to do it in a positive way and not as a frantic battering of yourself to 'get back to normal'. Every time it crosses your mind, on a breath out squeeze your tummy button towards your spine and pull all your lower abdominal muscles in. Every time you see one of the sticky stars in your house (see p. 41), do some pelvic floor squeezes. Every time you take the pram or buggy out, take a minute to stand in 'tadasana' or 'mountain pose' (p. 5) before you put your hands on the handle. Keep your shoulders relaxed as you walk along.

Head, neck and shoulders

EXERCISE FOR 14 DAYS – 3 MONTHS AFTER CHILDBIRTH

Feeding, lifting, carrying, doing all sorts of things with one hand while you hold your baby with the other, make it all too easy to build up knots of tension in your head, neck and shoulders. Ease them out with these stretches.

Sit cross-legged on the floor (if you have become supple in hips, knees and thighs, with all your ante-natal exercise, sit in half-lotus or lotus – one or both feet up on the opposite thigh). Stretch up your spine and the crown of your head, drop your shoulders, and close your eyes. You have been doing this for many months now. By slowing your breath down, stop your mind racing, and drop deep into the centre of yourself. Contact the deep core of yourself which you do not have much time to be aware of if you are rushing about or very tired. It's good, and moving, to know it's still there.

After a few minutes 'coming to centre', rub your hands together to warm them, then cup your face in your warm hands, separate your fingers, and blink your eyes open behind your hands. Allow your eyes to get used to the light, then float your hands slowly down into your lap.

Stand up in 'tadasana' or 'mountain pose' (see p. 5). Without letting your spine slump, on a breath out let your head fall forwards, stretch the back of your neck. Weight your head a little more by linking your hands and placing them on the back of your head, forearms lying along the sides of your face. Breathing steadily, hold the stretch for a few seconds. Breathing in, release your hands and float your head up to centre. On the breath out let the crown of your head fall backward, and stretch your throat. Continue through the usual sequence – stretching ear to shoulder each side, then twisting the neck to each side, then making slow head rolls. It's the same as you did before your baby was born, except now you are standing up instead of sitting, your spine lifting, hips firm, and abdomen scooped in.

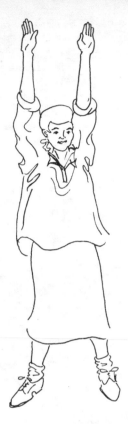

FIGURE 8.1

Arms stretched up

Stretch your shoulders this way. Breathe in, take your arms out at shoulder level, palms down. Breathing out, turn your palms up, feel your shoulders open, and stretch your arms above your head (Figure 8.1). Breathe in, and on the breath out stretch your right fingertips up a little further. Feel all the right side of your body stretch. On the breath in come back as you were. On the next breath out stretch your left fingertips up. Feel the left side of your body extend. Breathing in, relax. Stretch left and right sides alternately for six more breaths in and out. Then on a breath out stretch your arms out at shoulder level again.

Side and forward stretches

Stretch to the side in 'trikonasana' or 'triangle pose' (explained in detail on p. 6). Work both sides in this way. Next, stretch forwards in 'parsvottanasana' (explained in detail on p. 17). Let your lower back stretch and try to feel your whole back is flat and broad. While you are in this forward stretch, on a breath out pull your tummy muscles back towards your spine. They won't respond a lot at first, but little by little they get stronger.

Stride your feet wide apart and stretch forwards and then down – hands on the floor between your feet if you can, and then when you become even more supple, elbows to the floor (Figure 8.2). Hold the stretch for 20-30 seconds, breathing steadily, face and throat relaxed. On a breath out, come up.

FIGURE 8.2

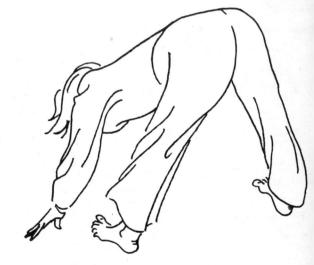

Forward, downward stretch

Exercises for abdominals and hips

After an ordinary birth it often takes 3 or 4 more weeks before you start to feel as though your abdominal muscles might have a life of their own again. Give them time. Persistent, gentle exercise will help them on their way.

Cat stretches

Coming on to all fours, arch and flatten your back half-a-dozen times, arching up on a breath out, flattening on a breath in. With each arch upwards scoop your abdominal muscles as flat up towards your spine as you can.

After half-a-dozen of these, separate your knees more and put your feet together. Breath in and breathing out, stretch your bottom down towards your feet, and your chest and face to the floor. In this stretch contract and release your pelvic floor muscles half-a-dozen times. Then breathe in, lift your head up and breathing out, walk your hands towards you and sit yourself up.

Lie down on your back and check that the centre line of your body is straight. Bend your knees up and separate your feet and knees a little. Link your hands behind your head. Inhale. Exhaling, bend your left elbow up to your right knee. Let the right foot come off the floor so the knee meets the elbow. Inhaling, relax down. Exhaling, take your right elbow to your left knee, let your left foot come off the floor. Inhaling, relax down. Exhaling, take your right elbow to your left knee; let your left foot come off the floor. Inhaling, relax down. Press your tummy muscles

FIGURE 8.3

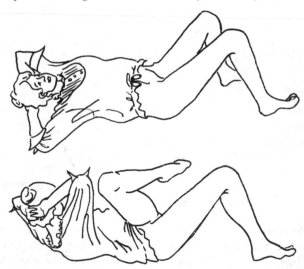

Diagonal elbow/knee sit ups, two types

back towards your spine as you do this – don't let them bulge out. Try eight repetitions each side to start with, and little by little, work up to twenty-four. There is nothing to be gained by overstressing your muscles doing twenty-four the first day (Figure 8.3).

After doing however many you decide to do on this particular day, hug your knees to your chest and relax.

Now place your feet back on the floor as they were before, and lie your arms down by your sides. Inhale. As you exhale push your hips up in the air. Inhaling, let them drop towards the floor but not on to it. Exhaling, push them up again. Inhaling, let them release down (Figure 8.4). Really notice your lower abdominal, buttock and thigh muscles working. Try eight times up and down with your hips at first. Gradually add on a couple more repetitions each day until you are up to twenty-four (unbelievable when you first try – but it gets easier). When you finish hug your knees to your chest again to let your back and tummy relax.

FIGURE 8.4

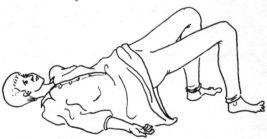

Bridge exercise

Now stretch your heels away; lie flat on the floor. On a breath out, press your abdomen towards your back and lift your feet vertically into the air. On a breath in stretch your legs wide apart; on the breath out bring your feet up to the centre and cross them at the ankles. Repeat this 'scissoring', apart on a breath in, together and crossing on a breath out, eight times at first, then add on a few more each day till you get to twenty-four. When you finish hug your knees to your chest again (Figure 8.5).

FIGURE 8.5

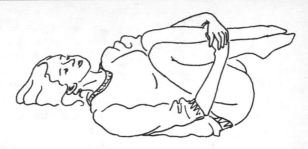

Hug knees to chest

Sitting poses

Don't lose all the extra stretch you've made in your thighs doing antenatal exercises. Sitting tall, stretch your legs wide apart. After 20-30 seconds, on a breath out, walk your hands forwards and extend your upper body forwards along the floor between your legs. Stay here, breathing steadily, for 20 seconds or so, then on a breath in lift your head up; on a breath out walk your hands back towards you and come up.

Bring the soles of your feet together and hold on to them. Relax your knees and thighs down towards the floor. If your thighs feel loose, stretch them even more by exhaling and making a forward bend with your upper body, keeping your back long. Aim to get your chin, rather than your forehead, on to the floor.

Alternate nostril breathing

Finish your session with this very relaxing breathing. It is useful for calming yourself down at any time – if you can't sleep, for instance. One woman recently told me she used it to calm herself down when her car broke down and she was waiting for the breakdown service. (What presence of mind!)

Sit yourself cross-legged, or if your hips, knees, and ankles have become very supple, sit in lotus pose, putting each foot up on the opposite thigh. Rest your left hand on your left knee. Put the third finger of your right hand on your forehead, just above the bridge of your nose, so that you can close your right nostril with your thumb and your left nostril with your fourth finger. Lift your spine and relax your shoulders. Exhale deeply.

Close your right nostril with your thumb, breathe in through your left nostril.

Close your left nostril with your fourth finger. Hold them both closed for a moment.

Release your right nostril and breathe out through the right. Breathe in through the right.

Close the right nostril with your thumb. Hold both closed for a moment.

Release your left nostril and breathe out through the left.

Carry on with this breathing, noticing how your breath gets deeper and slower. Experiment with closing your nostrils with lighter and lighter pressure so you aren't pushing your nose around.

After a few minutes, or whenever you feel you've had enough, slowly float your right hand down to your right knee, and take a few breaths to let your breathing come back to an everyday level.

Without disturbing yourself too much, lie down on your back for a few moments of deep relaxation. Starting with your feet and working your way up your body, become aware of each part of you, and on a breath out, let it go, until you are relaxed from your toes to the top of your head. Allow yourself some time of deep rest, sinking further and further into the floor, travelling in your imagination, if you like, to some favourite landscape and resting there.

Only when you feel like it, gradually become aware of the room again. Yawn, stretch, and curl up on your side for a few moments before pressing your hands into the floor and helping yourself up.

CO-COUNSELLING AND MASSAGE

We all need 'mothering' – including mothers – if what 'mothering' means is some tender and considerate attention especially for ourselves. Try to find some occasions, perhaps once a week with a friend, when you can give each other some 'mothering', such as 20 minutes or half-an-hour each of each other's exclusive attention to talk about anything that is on your mind, and also some time to give each other a massage – shoulder and back massage is specially useful – so that you're not doing all the giving that goes on around you. When your baby or babies get crawling or toddling this is hard to arrange during the day, but try to get together for a couple of hours in the evening instead.

CHAPTER 9

MOVING ON: 3 MONTHS AND ONWARDS

By the time your baby is 12 weeks old you will probably feel you have travelled some way from the experience of birth, and begun to reclaim your body, and work out, in many ways, how to let your baby and yourself be separate people, and both get as many as possible of the things you want in your life. You will have worked out all the manoeuvres of how to get to the shops or a friend's house, or to work, and got over the first intensities of panic, of feeling, perhaps for the first time, how dangerous the world is (traffic, guns, bombs) and how powerful your protective feelings towards this small person are.

If you've followed through the exercises in this book you are probably stronger, more supple, and more in touch with your body than you were. Perhaps you might like to go on developing these qualities in yourself, you might find it interesting to go on doing things which make you feel good about your body.

You might like to try one of the many martial arts. Great strength and confidence comes from learning self-defence and physical self-reliance. Many sports centres and women's groups run women-only classes if you prefer to work with women only.

Yoga classes are available almost everywhere. Ask around for a teacher who sounds as though she or he is on your wavelength. The balance between physical and spiritual varies a great deal from class to class and you may have a firm preference one way or another.

Look up dance centres in the phone book – if you are near a big city there are probably several within your reach. They will usually send you a brochure free of charge and you can compare cost and what's on offer. Women's centres often have a dance or movement class available as well. If you live in a small community watch the local press for advertisements for classes.

If you can't get a babysitter, or can't afford or don't fancy classes, you might have a friend who teaches movement who would work with a small group of you at your home in return for a small payment or something you can do for her. Alternatively, a small group could take it in turns to 'lead' an evening of exercise, stretching and breathing.

FIGURE 9.1

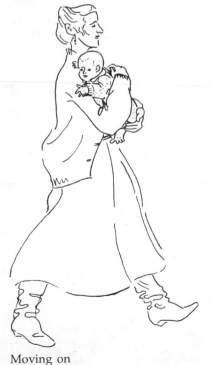

Moving on

Having a baby may have put you in touch with feelings and aspects of your personality of which you weren't aware before. If you want to grow and develop more in these ways, see what groups are on offer at your local women's centre (if you're not sure whether there is one, ask at the library) or set up your own group using *In Our Own Hands* by Sheila Ernst and Lucy Goodison (Women's Press, 1981), a lovely book full of ideas and starting-places for groups trying to explore thoughts and feelings.

Moving and being moved – both in the physical and emotional sense – can keep our lives from getting stuck, and keep us alive and growing. As your baby grows make sure you have some time and space for yourself as well – and keep moving on!

APPENDIX:
BIRTH REPORTS

1   Our baby was already a few days late. We indulged
in our own alternative 'prostaglandin treatment',
more fun than NHS pessaries – and in this case just
as effective!

At 4a.m. I got up for my obligatory pee, but I did
seem to have more backache than usual. I was also
sick.

At 5 a.m. I woke Michael since I thought that this
might be it. The gaps between contractions were not
of text book duration but difficult to assess, frequent
but short and irregular. I coped by moving around,
rocking, breathing and unleashing my vitriolic
tongue with assorted obscenities. On two or three
occasions I said 'Sod this, these bloody exercises
don't work at all. The minute I get there I'm having
an epidural and that's that.' Michael held me up,
rubbed my back, breathed with me, and just nodded
and smiled.

At 8a.m. I felt I couldn't stay at home any longer
so we bundled off in the car, me rolling around in
the back seat. We were put in a room straightaway
with the lovely white-haired Sister X whose back-
rubbing technique was quite incredible and when I
sheepishly babbled, 'I want an active birth but I
don't know if I can go through with it', she
reassured me and said, 'Let's see how things are
going, shall we?' Now came the good news. I was
7 cm dilated.

Unfortunately the liquor was meconium stained.
My membranes were ruptured which I agreed to
and a scalp electrode placed on my baby's head. I
had never liked the idea of scalp electrodes (rather a

nasty initiation to the outside world for a baby, I think) but I could see that it was justifiable in the case of fetal distress.

I used Entonox for transition, effective as pain relief, but it tended to make me feel a bit too stoned to be fully in control. Yes, transition is pretty tough. I got into some serious beanbag biting. I wanted to push, in fact my diaphragm was doing so involuntarily, and I must say that the knee/chest 'huff, huff, blow' honestly does work, although I spent so long doing it that I felt like a demented steam engine.

At 10.20a.m. I commenced pushing in a squatting position although later amended this to a supported squat. This part was absolutely marvellous, not painful at all, but quite an incredible feeling. At 10.53a.m. out he came! As his head was out Michael and I put our hands down to touch him and he actually looked up at us.

Our son spent his first few minutes yelling and screaming, so the meconium stained liquor was obviously nothing too much to worry about. Obviously I couldn't suckle him straightaway; he needed a stomach wash out and a quick once-over by the paediatricians, but they kept him in the room to do this so I could still see him. I resisted the offer of syntometrin to expel the placenta. When I got hold of the baby he suckled resolutely straightaway and the placenta and membranes slipped out easily, complete and intact.

Altogether it was a lovely labour and an overwhelming experience. All three of us felt marvellous. We all had a cuddle, then I got up and had a bath. It had taken just 7 hours in all, which I don't think is bad at all for a first 'go'.

Now on the post-natal ward I feel like I could play a squash tournament – really fit and healthy. I'm convinced that the exercise classes made me fitter physically, well-prepared mentally, and made my labour shorter and easier.

2 I was 2 weeks overdue and induction loomed up, bringing with it a feeling of disappointment and nervousness. This was my second child and I had really wanted to spend some of my labour at home with my little boy, hopefully feeling more relaxed and managing to cope with the contractions because of this. I had had to go to the hospital very early with my first child as my membranes ruptured before I started contracting. It had certainly made the labour seem longer and more arduous than I would have wanted. I had attended Paddy's classes this time in the hope that I could take a more active part in controlling my labour and the fact that I was to be induced made me feel that it was out of my hands once again.

As it turned out the whole labour and birth were a tremendous experience and I felt fully in control. I arrived at the labour ward ready for induction having had a good night's sleep, a lovely bath, and a big breakfast. It was a strange feeling driving to the hospital knowing that later that day I would be giving birth to our second child. I was excited but nervous.

I was examined by the doctor who felt that if my membranes were ruptured I would manage to get going without the help of drugs – that suited me and meant that I was able to move about. I had no pain at all for about half an hour and then I started contracting about every 10 minutes. I was walking up and down the corridors and not finding the pain too severe. We decided that Peter should go to the shops quickly as I obviously had some way to go.

He had only been gone about 15 minutes when the pains became stronger and more frequent. I continued to walk around, but was finding it difficult to concentrate on my breathing during the contractions. Twenty minutes later Peter returned to find me huffing and puffing and unable to really have a conversation. I was still up but finding that I needed to sit in the big armchair much more frequently. There seemed to be little or no breaks in between the contractions and I was beginning to think that I would need something to help me cope if this was to carry on for a couple of hours. The midwife asked me to climb back on to the bed to check the baby's heartbeat. It was all I could do to walk from the chair to the bed. I used the rocking movement which had helped me throughout the labour as I leaned on the bed. There was a strange feeling in my bottom the next contraction, and I got a strong urge to push. I still had not got on to the bed! The midwife did a quick vaginal examination once I was on the bed and then told me to push as hard as I could. After five hard pushes the head was delivered swiftly followed by some large shoulders and we then had 10lbs of baby boy on my tummy! The labour was over – I couldn't believe it. It had taken 1 hour 40 minutes from beginning to end. I felt great although I had an attack of the shivers for about 20 minutes.

Looking back, induction was the only interference I had and the labour afterwards was as natural as possible. Our baby is a relaxed, contented fellow and I'm sure that is partly because I was not too exhausted after a long and painful labour. Paddy's exercises both during the labour and afterwards have been very easy to do and very helpful. I hope that others who end up being induced find that they have a fulfilling experience too.

3   Somewhere between 8 and 9am I noticed my 'Braxton Hicks' contractions were rather regular, 5-10 minutes apart but not painful. I had not had a 'show' and my membranes were intact so I chose to ignore them. At about midday I was queuing in Mothercare(!) to buy some baby things when I felt the contractions were getting decidedly uncomfortable and wished I could get down and sway my hips. But I still did not believe I could be in labour, after all it was 2 weeks early, and I expected to be at least a week late.

On coming out of Mothercare my toddler demanded a wee so we went to the public loos. I went too and there was my 'show', albeit rather insignificant – pink/brown streak of blood on the loo paper. Perhaps I am in labour, I thought.

We reached home and it was bliss to be able to kneel and sway my hips with contractions which by now were coming every 3 minutes.

In between contractions I got my bag ready, arranged for a friend to have my little girl, and had some lunch. I then had difficulty getting off the loo because of diarrhoea – which made me think, either I'm not in labour and I've got a tummy bug, or I'm going to have the baby in the loo!

We made it to the hospital by 2p.m., by which time I had great difficulty controlling myself in the car because I was sat up. I had to keep moving during contractions and was desperate to get back on to all fours.

The pain was intense and I was afraid of being told I wasn't dilating as I knew I would repeat my performance of my first labour and panic and demand an epidural if nothing had happened by then.

'Eureka!' – I was 6 cm dilated with a thin stretchy cervix. I squatted on the pillows between contractions and rested, then when the contraction came I wanted to go on all fours. I couldn't bear to be touched, – even Paul or the midwife rubbing my back wasn't right. I held my tummy myself which eased the feeling a bit.

I tried some gas and air, but I felt that I lost control while I was using it, and so even though without it I was thrashing about, biting the beanbag and making an awful racket, I carried on without!

As I approached the second stage the pain moved to my back: so much so that I thought it would break. I screamed for someone to take the backache away, but I still didn't want it rubbed.

I had taken my gown off because it was too hot and in the way, and I was on all fours over a beanbag. I tried to sit back and squat to push, but I couldn't because of the backache – so on all fours, the way I had sworn I would not deliver, I pushed and shouted and shouted and pushed!

My son was born an hour and a half after I'd reached hospital! I didn't need stitches either!

I am glad I did it on my own this time. I feel I achieved what I hoped, but did not believe I could.

Being on all fours had its drawback in that I could not see my baby emerging from me or hold him as he was delivered, but at the time I couldn't have cared less. It seemed ages though until he was brought for me to see and hold, but it was in fact only seconds.

4 Sunday 14th April. Baby due. Feel like an overblown flower but less good looking. Nothing happened. Strip the wallpaper in the dining room. Nothing happened.

Monday 15th: Mum says baby will arrive today, her coral wedding anniversary. Nothing happened.

Tuesday 16th: Took Chris to school. Went to the shops, bought food for week. Hung out first lot of washing. Collected Chris from school. Did two more lots of washing. Workmen took down door to kitchen. Cooked dinner with secret ingredient brick dust.

10.30p.m. Go to bed

10.32p.m. Ping. Out of bed into loo very fast. Waters had broken. Wake Chris and send him to my sister.

11.15p.m. Arrive hospital.

11.45p.m. Put on monitor for 20-minute trace. Strong contractions and baby's heartbeat good.

12.00p.m.-4.00a.m. went to loo four times, was sick twice. Walked around, lay down, squatted on beanbag, as the mood took me. Also listened to tape on my headset. Pain in the top of my left leg every time I passed a motion. Midwives still can't feel how the baby is laying because I am so tight.

4.00a.m.-7.00a.m. Contractions every 3 minutes but it hurts more if I try to move at all. I do my breathing and watch the clock.

7.30a.m. I need some help, I am worn out. Try gas and air – not much help but it gives me something to do. I have reached 10 cm. They ask me to start to push. I am on the bed sat up.

8.00a.m. Every contraction I push and get cramp in my leg. Oh dear.

9.30a.m. I am still pushing but they say I can rest as I am getting nowhere. My body says you will push. More people arrive to examine me.

10.00a.m. This child has its head sideways – he will not come out like that. Spinal injection.

10.45a.m. feet numb, put in stirrups. Oh pain. I wish they were using the forceps on my feet. They must push the baby back up, turn him and pull him out.

11.00a.m. I can feel him being born – head, shoulders and legs. It's a boy. The birth witnessed by twelve strangers but I was an interesting case. I have taught the students a lot.

18th April 11a.m. allowed to sit up. 12.30 walk unaided to bathroom and have a bath. Feel very good, stitches a bit sore but I am upright and walking better than most.

21st April. Told by fellow patient to stop bouncing around and looking so fit, but another said it inspired them to see how quickly you can recover.

It is now 3 weeks later. I am in my normal clothes and doing a normal day's work. Thank you Paddy for all your help.

5 It rained and there was thunder and much lightning all night. We were fully awake by 3 a.m., soon after which I felt my first contraction, and within 10 minutes another, just like a period pain. I breathed through each and I could feel myself going with the feeling. The contractions increased in intensity quite quickly, and I varied positions according to the amount of pain, either standing, rocking, swaying my hips or kneeling over a seat. I telephoned labour ward at 5.30a.m. to tell them I would be visiting later on. I was advised to wait until contractions were regular – every 5 minutes for an hour.

Jim made tea and we slowly got organized. At 6a.m. contractions were coming every 5 minutes. Now I needed much more help from Jim to keep me breathing, which I did very, very slowly and deeply. He rubbed my back and timed contractions. I found contractions easiest on all fours or leaning over a seat, letting myself moan and croon. I also found relief sitting with my back to Jim, on his knees with my knees wide apart. This way he could hold my sides and help me sway side to side.

At 7a.m. we phoned the labour ward – an hour of regular contractions. We were advised to have breakfast, take a bath, since first babies don't arrive very quickly.

While I was in the bath I must have passed into second stage as pushing contractions started. I didn't really recognize what was happening, although I did pant, rather than breathe, through the contractions. When I got out of the bath I realized what the situation was and decided to give breakfast a miss! The car ride was quite relaxing but a bit frightening when contractions came. Would I make it? I had a feel and there was no head! I was worried that my waters had not broken, but of course I realize now they must have broken in the bath and I had not noticed.

I asked for room 3 and told sister I was pushing. I immediately shed all my clothes – this felt more comfortable and most natural. I crawled on to the bed and tried to tell sister that I wanted to deliver squatting.

Everything was happening so fast. I really didn't have time to plan my next move. I felt a bit flustered. Anyway, it was announced that I was fully dilated, and the rest was up to me. Help – what did she mean? I soon found out – pushing into my bottom – I had had no idea just how hard I would have to push.

Oh, what pain! I thought I was getting nowhere

but everyone encouraged me. They could see the baby's hair and it was black. Poor sister was nearly lying down waiting for the head. She told me to pant and the baby's head was born – more like a rugby ball than a grapefruit! Great excitement; sister asked me to help her by catching the baby's shoulders as he came out. All arms and legs, very alert and crying – and he wasn't the only one. I pulled baby on to my tummy. How absolutely wonderful. We had done it. Jim and I were ecstatic.

The third stage was completed and we marvelled at the placenta which had sustained this tiny life for 9 months.

I was washed and felt really spoilt. Sister and her team had done everything we had wanted and asked for in our active birth. They had been truly fantastic.

6 [Suzanne was brought into hospital after having been 4 cm dilated for several days, with no other signs of impending labour.]

I agreed to have my waters broken. I don't know why really. Everybody was so kind and super it disarmed me if I can put it that way. I knew once this was done we were committed to delivering this baby somehow that day. My waters were broken at 11.15 and by 1.15 very little had happened. I was getting very upset as sister said that they would have to use cyntocinon if something did not happen in another couple of hours. Luckily that threat did the trick, and after a few plies and stretch exercises my contractions started – every 5 minutes. I was progressing very nicely but by 5 to 3 I was only 5 cm dilated. I said 'That's it. No more. Epidural.' (Told you I was a coward.) I could not bear another several hours of that pain without much progress. It seems my body reacts well to such crisis points, as from then on – wham – I was dilating again (still screaming for my epidural). [When she realized that she was dilating fast she decided not to have the epidural.]

Up to transition I got through my contractions leaning on a chair and rocking my hips which was great. I used my breathing quite efficiently and when I got to the stage of 'bugger this I want to go home' sister made me concentrate on my breathing which kept me relatively calm. I used gas and air for the transition stage very successfully. I was allowed to push at 3.45. I delivered semi-squatting – I started off each push in a squat and ended up in a floppy heap at the end of the bed. When I got to the unbearable phase I remembered the baby. I felt so sorry for her and it made me stop complaining. I asked them not to cut me and I only tore a little – two small stitches were needed. Sylvia [her baby] sucked immediately and I had a cup of tea and a bath. It was wonderful, I felt so healthy, drug-free and normal, what a difference from last time. Thank God I didn't have the epidural or anything else. It was so exciting and let's face it, it's got to hurt if it means anything to you.

7 4.30p.m. We arrive at hospital. I feel a bit sheepish, thinking that they'll probably send me home and tell me to come back when I'm really in labour. They have a low bed waiting for me and two beanbags. I have a midwife and a student midwife who both seem keen on active births. Great! Internal examination. Baby's head is well down and I am 6 cm dilated. YIPPEE! This *is* it! They decide to break my waters, to speed things up, and the contractions certainly did start to get very powerful. I barely got a break in between them, but they were still very easy to cope with by using the deep breathing and kneeling up to rock. I alternated between hanging round Paul's neck (so he could rub my back) and kneeling forwards on to cushions and a beanbag which were piled up on to the head of the bed. In between it was nice to crash out either forwards or sideways on to the pillows which felt wonderfully cool. Paul also held a very cold flannel against the base of my spine which felt wonderful. I felt progressively more and more instinctual and my body completely took control over my mind. I was making a lot of noises, moaning and sighing, which seemed to come very naturally and helped enormously. At about 6.20 I suddenly wanted to push. The midwives were very encouraging and kind – even when I lost control in a couple of the contractions. The pushing sensation had taken me so much by surprise that I had spent a few contractions wailing 'No! no! I can't do it!' With a bit of helpful encouragement, though, I found that I could do it and I began to really enjoy the sensations of the head descending. I found it really exhilarating – it is probably the best experience I will ever have. The baby's head was born and the body was turned and then slithered out very easily. A boy! I was surprised as I'd convinced myself I'd have a little girl. Nevertheless I was delighted. Paul was beside himself and I had never felt so good. I took the baby on to my stomach. He was very alert and absolutely gorgeous. I suckled him straightaway and he seemed very strong. I got up after about an hour and a half and had a bath which was lovely.

8 [This was Sally's second baby. She came into hospital in the early evening when she had been having contractions every 5 minutes for a couple of hours. However, an internal examination revealed that her cervix was still only effacing, not dilated at all. 'Feeling foolish', Sally and her husband Steve went back home, but could not sleep, so stayed awake chatting and playing a game. Later that night. . . .]

As we played contractions began again and were strong enough to have to do something about them. I found holding on to the chest of drawers, bent at the hips and swivelling about very comfortable. As soon as I got into that position any pain or discomfort seemed to vanish. The other thing that was very useful was to kneel on the floor with my body over a pile of pillows on the bed, and again moving the hips was very useful. Towards midnight contractions were coming very quickly. Steve went to phone the hospital. I stood on the stairs saying, 'I'm sure this is more than every 5 minutes', and he stood in the hall with the phone in his hand saying, 'Go and get dressed, go and get dressed! When I got to the bedroom again I felt I could hardly stand, and wonder how I got out of my nightie and into my clothes. Somehow I got down the stairs and into the car.

We had agreed I would travel in the back, and we pushed forward the front passenger seat so that I could get on the floor if I wanted. Quite frankly I didn't know what I wanted. I spent the time crawling about up and down the back seat, always on all fours, and I remember clearly clutching the back of the front seat begging Steve not to drive so fast. He drove mostly with one hand, the other hand massaging my back, which was a great help. Of course, all the traffic lights were against us!

I was frightened at this point, and I felt quite out of control. I couldn't get comfortable, and there didn't seem to be any pause in what was happening to me. I had an image of being in a very high sea, clinging to a piece of wood with waves that threw the log high and then plunged it deep in between them. I felt most alone at this point because Steve was worried about getting to the safety of the hospital. It was useful to have considered in class beforehand what it might be like to be frightened, even though it was worse than I had projected. I think I do like to be in control of myself, and felt at this point that I was being thrown about and taken over by forces greater than me.

When we arrived at the hospital I really could hardly walk properly down the corridor. A quick lean on the reception counter was helpful. Sister helped me into the delivery room. I undressed and put on the gown. I can honestly say I didn't feel pain but did feel overwhelming waves that seemed to be in my head. I felt shaky and sick and I really wanted to crawl into a dark corner.

I was 9 cm dilated. I got up on all fours and Steve stood at the end of the bed and I pushed my head into him. This was tremendously comforting. I felt that he was like a rock, a still point in an experience that was threatening to overwhelm me. Inevitably I had to turn round eventually and I used the pillows to support me until the student midwife brought me a beanbag, which I sprawled over and found very comfortable.

When the urge to push came I was amazed at the power and insistence of the desire. I seemed to be able to breathe successfully through the desire to push. [Sally's midwife at this point tried to give her some gas and air.] I pushed the mask aside and puff puff blowed which was more successful. The time to push came and I made a great deal of noise. I didn't enjoy pushing very much because I was told to give three pushes with each contraction and I felt I couldn't catch enough breath to do this. My feeling was that I should push more calmly and slowly and not worry about the third push. Then I heard the midwife say that I would have to get on my side. I heard the panic in her voice and later Steve told me that at that point her hands were shaking. So go on my side I did. I remember looking down and seeing my bulging perineum. I was given an episiotomy to prevent a third degree tear. I did not feel the cut at all.

I didn't see the baby's head born, but I did see him as his body slithered free and I was filled with relief and admiration for what seemed this dignified and gentle baby. 'It's a boy', someone said, and somehow I thought of the Knights of the Round Table and their chivalry. He was placed across my thigh and he seemed very wonderful and I felt great respect for him somehow. As the lights were dimmed and deflected he opened his eyes. I felt wonderful and very fit and well and delighted.

FURTHER READING

Active Birth, Janet and Arthur Balaskas,
New Life, Janet and Arthur Balaskas, Sidgwick &
Jackson, 1979.
Both books discuss the physiology and psychology
of 'active birth' and suggest programmes of exercise
for healthy pregnancy and active labour.

Exercises for Childbirth, Barbara Dale and Johanna
Roeber, Century, 1982.
Sensitive book describing a group of exercises to
stretch and tone the body and a loving philosophy
of birth.

Yoga and Pregnancy, Sophie Hoare
Precise and perceptive account of the application of
yoga practice in pregnancy.

Pregnancy and Childbirth, Sheila Kitzinger, Michael
Jackson, 1980.
A well indexed mine of information, clearly illus-
trated and firmly woman-centred in its approach.

Birth Over Thirty, Sheila Kitzinger, Sheldon Press,
1982.
Just the thing for those of us who are.

Woman's Experience of Sex, Sheila Kitzinger, Dorling
Kindersley, 1983. Extremely useful support, advice,
information about sex in pregnancy, the sexuality of
birth, sex after birth, and managing episiotomy or
Caesarian wounds, in the relevant chapters of this
book.

Birth Reborn, Michel Odent, Souvenir Press, 1984.
Describes birth practices in the famous Pithiviers

clinic. Lovely photographs, inspiring text.

Entering the World, Michel Odent, Marion Boyars, 1984.
A philosophical discussion of Odent's approach to birth.

Your Body, Your Baby, Your Life, Angela Phillips, Pandora Press, 1983.
A thorough and dynamic book which gives information on all aspects of pregnancy and birth, and life with a small baby.

From Here to Maternity, Ann Oakley, Pelican, 1979.
Interviews with women throughout their pregnancies and the months after birth. A wealth of shared experience.

In Labour: Women and Power in the Birthplace, Barbara Katz Rothman, Junction Books 1982.
Exciting book which analyses clearly how the language and practice of maternity care has taken power away from women and midwives during the 1970s, and describing the growth of these women's struggle to get that power back.

Postnatal Exercises, Barbara Whiteford and Margie Polden, Century, 1984.
Sound ideas for the gradual strengthening of your body after your baby's birth.

INDEX

DISCOVERING WOMEN'S HISTORY
A Practical Manual

by Deirdre Beddoe
'An invaluable and fascinating guide to the raw
material for anyone approaching this unexplored
territory.'

The Sunday Times

0-86358-008-4   232pp   illustrated

ON YOUR OWN
A Guide for Independent Women

by Jean Shapiro
A bible for all divorced and widowed women,
covering all of the practical and emotional matters
that women are likely to face when they find
themselves suddenly 'on their own'.
0-86358-027-0c   250pp   illustrated
        045-9p

NATURAL HEALING IN GYNECOLOGY
A User's Guide

by Rina Nissim
'. . . compels us to care for our health in an intelligent
and truly preventive manner. It provides a range of
healing alternatives from Eastern and Western
cultures, and critiques the limits of conventional
Western medicine, giving us the power of
choice. . . An unusual and valuable resource indeed.'
        Boston Women's Health Book Collective
086358 063 7c   192pp   illustrated
086358 069 6p